Sport Medicine: Incidence & Treatment of Athletic Injuries

A Volume in MSS' series on Sport Medicine

Papers by
E. C. Percy, Robert L. Larson, Thomas R. Peterson et al.

MSS Information Corporation
655 Madison Avenue, New York, N.Y. 10021

Library of Congress Cataloging in Publication Data
Main entry under title:

Sport medicine.

.A collection of articles previously published in
various journals.
   1.   Sport--Accidents and injuries--Addresses, essays,
lectures.   I.   Percy, E. C.   [DNLM: 1.   Athletic
injuries--Collected works.   2.   Sport medicine--
Collected works.   QT260 S7637   1973]
RD131.S76   617'.1027   73-10382
ISBN   0-8422-7142-2

TABLE OF CONTENTS

CREDITS AND ACKNOWLEDGEMENTS

Aronson, Neal I., "Head and Neck Injuries in Athletes," *Maryland Medical Journal,* 1967, 16:59-65.

Blazina, Martin E., "Shoulder Injuries in Athletics," *Journal of the American College Health Association,* 1966, 15:143-145.

Botton, Jacques E., "Athletic Head and Spinal Injuries," *Virginia Medical Monthly,* 1969, 96:79-84 *passim.*

Burry, Hugh C., "Late Effects of Neglected Soft Tissue Injury," *Proceedings of the Royal Society of Medicine,* 1969, 62:930-932.

Cooperman, E.M.; J. Hogg; and W.M. Thurlbeck, "Mechanisms of Death in Shallow-water Scuba Diving," *Canadian Medical Association Journal,* 1968, 99:1128-1131.

Corrigan, A.B., "Rehabilitation of Injured Football Players," *The Medical Journal of Australia,* 1967, 1:441-442.

Devas, M.B., "Stress Fractures in Athletes," *Journal of the Royal College of General Practitioners,* 1970, 19:34-38.

Fekete, John F., "Severe Brain Injury and Death following Minor Hockey Accidents: The Effectiveness of the 'Safety Helmets' of Amateur Hockey Players," *The Canadian Medical Association Journal,* 1968, 99:1234-1239.

Froimson, Avrum I., "Tennis Leg," *Journal of the American Medical Association,* 1969, 209:415-416.

Froimson, Avrum I., "Treatment of Tennis Elbow with Forearm Support Band," *The Journal of Bone and Joint Surgery,* 1971, 53A:183-184.

Gardner, Richard C., "Tennis Elbow: Diagnosis, Pathology, and Treatment: Nine Severe Cases Treated by a New Reconstructive Operation," *Chemical Orthopaedics and Related Research,* 1970, No. 72:248-253.

Golding, D.N., "Real Tennis Elbow," *British Medical Journal,* 1968, 1:317.

Kirkman, N.F., "Mountain Accidents and Mountain Rescue in Great Britain," *British Medical Journal,* 1966, 1:162-164.

Kirkman, N.F.; and M.K. Hartley, "Mountain Accidents," *British Medical Journal,* 1968, 4:703.

Larson, Robert L., "Knee Injuries in the Adolescent Athlete," *Medical Times,* 1968, 96:679-688.

Newman, P.H.; J.P.S. Thomson; J.M. Barnes; and T.M.C. Moore, "A Clinic for Athletic Injuries," *Proceedings of the Royal Society of Medicine,* 1969, 62:939-941.

O'Hanlan, J. Treacy, "The Fosbury Flop," *Virginia Medical Monthly,* 1968, 95:717-719.

Paterson, Dennis C.; and John G. Sweeney, "Power-boat Injuries to Swimmers," *Medical Journal of Australia*, 1968, 2:1090-1092.

Percy, E.C., "The Snowmobile: Friend or Foe?," *The Journal of Trauma*, 1972, 12: 444-446.

Percy, E.C.; R.O. Hill; and J.E. Callaghan, "The 'Sprained' Ankle," *The Journal of Trauma*, 1969, 9:972-986.

Peterson, Thomas R., "The Cross-body Block, the Major Cause of Knee Injuries," *Journal of the American Medical Association*, 1970, 211:449-452.

Rowe, Murle Laurens, "Varsity Football: Knee and Ankle Injury," *New York Journal of Medicine*, 1969, 69:3000-3003.

Rylander, C. Roy, "Rehabilitation of the Injured Athlete," *Delaware Medical Journal*, 1969, 41:271-273.

Schuman, Stanley H., "Skateboard Injuries in a Campus Community," *Clinical Pediatrics*, 1967, 6:252-254.

Simurda, M.A., "Retrosternal Dislocation of the Clavicle: A Report of Four Cases and a Method of Repair," *The Canadian Journal of Surgery*, 1968, 11:487-490.

Stiles, Merritt H., "Medical Aspects of Skiing," *The Journal of the Maine Medical Association*, 1971, 62:136-138.

Weseley, Martin S.; and Philip A. Barenfeld, "Ball Throwers' Fracture of the Humerus: Six Case Reports," *Clinical Orthopaedics and Related Research*, 1969, 64:153-156.

Zinovieff, A., "Evaluation of the Results of Treatment of Soft Tissue Injury," *Proceedings of the Royal Society of Medicine*, 1969, 62:928-930.

PREFACE

In this era of strong emphasis on physical fitness, injuries associated with athletic activities have increased. Athletic injuries must therefore be thoroughly understood by physician and layman alike.

The most current methods of treatment for athletic injuries are considered in this MSS volume in the Sport Medicine Series. Among the topics covered are "sprained" ankles, knee injuries in adolescents, tennis elbow and tennis leg, fractures of the humerus, shoulder injuries, fatal brain injuries resulting from hockey, stress fractures, and soft tissue injuries. The medical dangers of skiing, snowmobiles, skateboards, boating and scuba diving are also discussed.

Incidence & Treatment of Athletic Injuries

THE "SPRAINED" ANKLE

E. C. PERCY, M.D., F.A.C.S., F.R.C.S.(C), R. O. HILL, M.D., AND
J. E. CALLAGHAN, M.D.

The purpose of this paper is to discuss a preliminary report of a more realistic approach to the diagnosis and subsequent treatment of the so-called "sprained" ankle. In this study, contrast dye arthrography has been employed to differentiate minor injuries from the seriously disrupted ankle. A classification of soft tissue injuries to the lateral aspect of the ankle is put forward, and a method of treatment based on the arthrographic findings is proposed. Mobilization only is recommended for the minor injuries, and immobilization for the partial tears of the lateral structures. Surgical repair is advocated for the completely disrupted ankle.

HISTORICAL REVIEW

Probably the commonest injury involving a joint is the lesion described as a simple inversion sprain of the ankle, resulting from what the layman describes as "turning his ankle." The term "ankle sprain" is as inaccurate a diagnosis as is that of a "broken leg." The lesion is generally by no means simple, and is quite often more than a sprain. Indeed. as DeVries (15) notes, the frequent observation that a severe ankle sprain is often worse than a fracture may well be true if treatment is inadequate. A fracture is readily recognized radiologically, so that appropriate treatment in the form of plaster casting or open reduction can be instituted at once. If, on the other hand, X-rays show no evidence of bony damage, the whole injury is dismissed as "only a sprain." The treatment applied at this stage varies with the whims of the treating physician. It may consist of injection of local anesthetic (28, 32), simple adhesive or elastic bandaging (19, 20, 40), plaster casting, or even operative repair of the torn soft tissues (1, 2, 5, 6, 7, 13, 31, 37, 39, 41). If plaster casting is employed, the duration of immobilization varies considerably, recommendations in the literature varying from 3 to 10 weeks in a below-knee walking cast (8, 12, 15, 36).

Bonnin (4, 5), who in the past has recommended conservatism, more recently recommends surgical repair for young active people whose ankles show evidence of instability. Clark et al. (9) reviewed patients treated in the Canadian Armed Services and reported similar results from operative repair and casting alone. They concluded that surgical repair should be carried out in young active adults only. Freeman (19), on the other hand, feels that all ruptures of the lateral ligament of the ankle should be treated by mobilization. Many surgeons in the past,

Presented at the Twenty-eighth Annual Session of the American Association for the Surgery of Trauma, Montreal, Quebec, October 18–20, 1968.

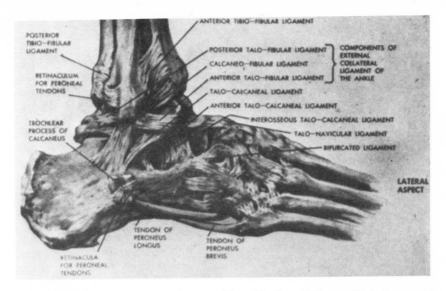

FIG. 1. The anatomy of the lateral aspect of the ankle. From F. Netter, Clinical symposia, Vol. 18, No. 1, 1966, (C) CIBA.

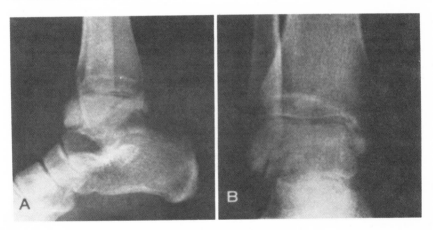

FIG. 2. A. Lateral arthrogram of normal ankle. B. A. P. arthrogram of normal ankle.

however, have carried out X-ray stress or inversion studies in the severe sprain (3, 4, 10, 16, 19, 28, 29, 35, 38). When gross instability has been demonstrated radiologically, some have recommended direct surgical repair, while others still recommend conservative treatment by plaster casting.

ANATOMY

Most sprains, occurring as they do in inversion, injure the lateral structures of the ankle joint. The lateral ligament is composed of three bands, each being quite

11

distinct from the others and serving a different functional role. The work of Leonard (34) and Brostrom (6) has done much to improve our knowledge of the functional role of these structures (Fig. 1).

The anterior band, referred to as the anterior talo-fibular ligament, runs from the anterior border of the lateral malleolus forward and medially to the neck of the talus. It lies deep and is fused with the capsule, and is taut in full equinus. It is the band most commonly injured in sprains, most sprains occurring in equinus. In this position the narrowest portion of the talus is in the mortise, and the ankle joint is physiologically less stable.

The posterior talo-fibular ligament runs from the bottom of the malleolar fossa medially and slightly backwards to the upper surface of the posterior tubercle of the talus. It also lies deep and fused to the capsule, but is taut in full dorsiflexion. It is probably infrequently torn in inversion sprains, occurring generally as they do in equinus, less commonly in the neutral position. No tears of this structure were noted in our series.

The middle portion, the calcaneo-fibular ligament, is a discrete narrow band lying superficial to the capsule, being separate from this latter structure. It runs from the tip of the lateral malleolus downwards and slightly backwards to the middle of the lateral surface of the calcaneum, a little above and behind the peroneal tubercle. It is probably taut at about 90°, and is functionally the most important of the three bands.

Note also in Figure 1 the superior peroneal retinaculum, which can be torn as an isolated entity in an inversion sprain.

The lateral talo-calcaneal ligament possibly plays a significant role in the symptom complex of the chronic unstable ankle. Occasionally it may be torn in the severe inversion sprain along with the calcaneo-fibular ligament, contributing perhaps to subtalar instability. The authors believe that by direct repair of the calcaneo-fibular ligament both the ankle joint and the subtalar joint are stabilized. No doubt subtalar instability does play a role in the unstable ankle. Freeman (20, 21, 22, 23), who has done extensive clinical investigation as well as studies on the experimental animal, feels that the unstable ankle results from a proprioceptive defect. He believes that the normal reflex coordination of muscle tone in posture and movement is disordered in the presence of capsular lesions in joints.

PROCEDURE

The major problem in the diagnostic assessment of "sprains" is in estimating the severity and nature of the lesion. Frequently in a severe inversion injury the dramatic swelling makes accurate assessment of the lesion difficult or impossible, unless there is gross instability in the ankle joint. The universally used method of assessment of integrity of the lateral structures of the ankle is forced inversion X-ray studies. Because of local discomfort and peroneal muscle spasm, accurate assessment of the talar tilt usually requires the use of local or general anesthetic. To ensure accuracy further, stress films should be taken at 90° and in full equinus, as will be demonstrated. To elucidate the picture further, X-rays in similar positions should be taken of the normal ankle for comparison. However, a tilt on the

12

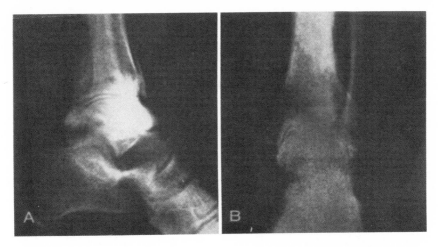

Fig. 3. A. Lateral X-ray, Type I tear. B. A.P. X-ray, Type I tear.

normal side, whether congenital or due to previous trauma and an unstable ankle, may confuse the whole picture. St. Jacques and Laurin (38) have reported the so-called normal talar tilt in children to vary from 0° to 27°.

An alternate method of assessment of severity of trauma of the lateral structures of the ankle following inversion sprains has now been in use at The Montreal General Hospital for the past 3 years. This method relies on the radiological assessment of the continuity of the joint with the use of a contrast dye, standard X-rays having excluded a fracture. Routine AP, lateral, and both oblique views are taken after the dye has been injected. We emphasize that this arthrogram should be done as soon as possible after the injury, although some slight mild local discomfort, due presumably to irritation of the dye, has been noted in the first 24 hours. Delay in carrying out this examination may allow filling of the defect with clots and fibrin formation and confuse the picture. We have used a solution of 30% Renografin® injected into the joint on the antero-medial aspect of the ankle, away from the site of the lesion. Any blood or fluid is of course aspirated prior to injecting the dye. In the ankle with an intact synovium and capsule, an average of 5 ml of solution can be injected into the joint. Some degree of discomfort is experienced by the patient at this point, and there is a mechanical resistance to the injection. In the case of previous injury with a healed but lax synovium and capsule, up to 15 ml can be injected. If a tear of the capsule is present, the injection can be done with ease, and amounts as large as 20 ml injected. In the normal ankle the synovium is as shown on the X-rays (Fig. 2). Note the natural capsular recesses in the AP and lateral projections which are well defined.

RESULTS

In a Type I tear the lesion resulting is a tear of the anterior capsule, and this is represented by a small leak or blow-out appearance on the anterior aspect of the

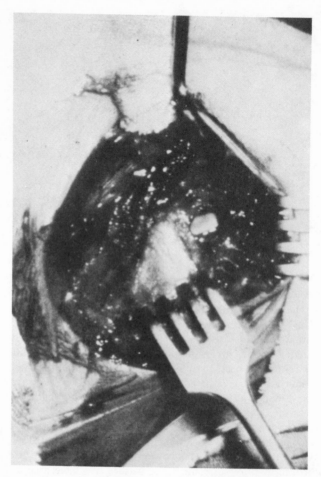

FIG. 4. Demonstrating small tear in anterior capsule in type I tear.

ankle joint (Fig. 3). Note that the escape of dye is anterior, with its flame-shaped appearance, and note also that the lateral structures are intact. The operative picture demonstrates a lesion of this type (Fig. 4). This was the first and only one of such lesions treated by operation in this series. (In all operative pictures which follow, the heel is on the left, and the forefoot is on the right. The operative incision is curved below the lateral malleolus as in Figure 5.) We feel that the treatment of such lesions should consist of mobilization only: that is, supportive measures on a symptomatic basis.

Type II tear results when the lesion is more extensive and the escape of dye is much more massive, and is seen both laterally and anteriorly (Fig. 6). Note the flame-shaped appearance of the escaped dye lying partially anterior and partially lateral. Figure 7 shows a tear of this type with rupture of the anterior capsule and

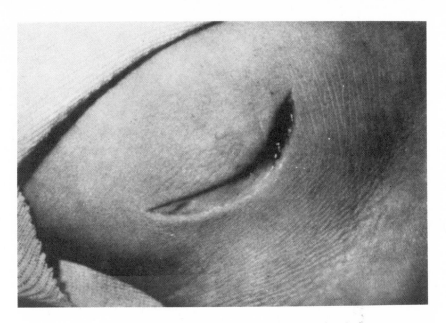

FIG. 5. Demonstrating operative incision below lateral maleolus.

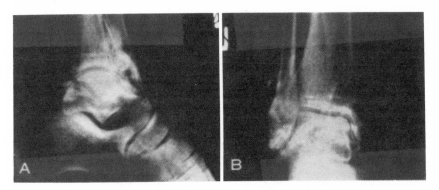

FIG. 6. A. Lateral X-ray, Type II tear. B. A.P. X-ray, Type II tear.

anterior talo-fibular ligament. Figure 8 demonstrates that, with the foot in the neutral position, the talus is stable in the ankle joint and cannot be subluxated. In equinus, however, as shown in Figure 9, the talus and foot can be internally rotated in the mortise, and with inversion the talus will subluxate. We feel that such lesions should probably be treated by immobilization in a below-knee walking cast for approximately 6 weeks. This capsular tear will no doubt heal anatomically with this treatment. The anterior talo-fibular ligament is intimately a portion of this structure, and should result in no residual laxity (11).

In the Type III tear the arthrogram shows (Fig. 10) massive escape of dye,

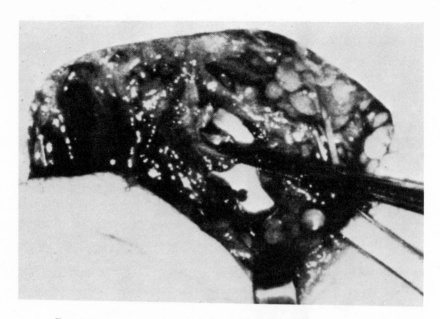

FIG. 7. Type II tear, forceps holding anterior talo-fibular ligament.

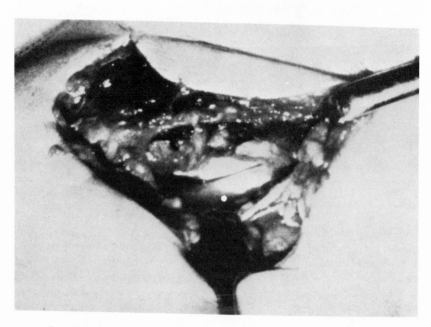

FIG. 8. Foot in neutral position, talus stable with inversion stress.

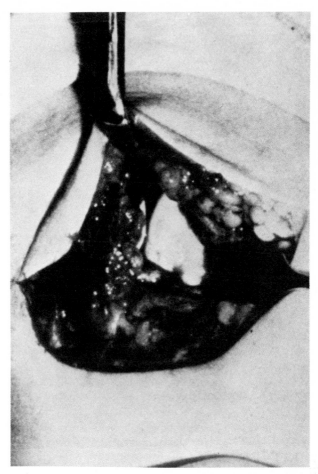

FIG. 9. Talus unstable in equinus. With internal rotation and inversion talus will sub-luxate.

demonstrating complete disruption of the antero-lateral structures. Note that most of the escape is lateral. In Figure 11 we see the anterior talo-fibular ligament and the calcaneo-fibular ligament which is detached from the os calcis, as it was invariably in our series. In such cases the talus will subluxate in both neutral and equinus positions (Fig. 12). This type of injury, in our opinion, demands surgical repair. We effect repair by suture of the capsule and direct suture of the calcaneo-fibular ligament to the periosteum at the original site of its attachment. We have immobilized these injuries postoperatively for 6 weeks in a below-knee cast, non-weight bearing for the first 2 weeks. Our plan of treatment parallels that suggested by Anderson et al. (1, 2) and by Elmslie (17).

An inversion injury which caused an isolated tear of the superior peroneal retinaculum demonstrated the following arthrographic findings as seen in Figure

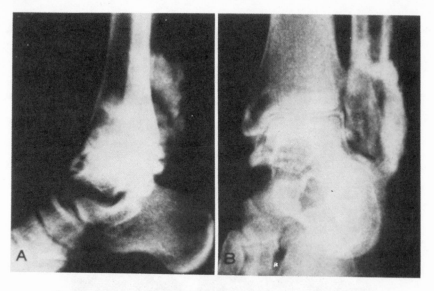

FIG. 10. A. Lateral X-ray, Type III tear. B. A.P. X-ray, Type III tear.

13. The escape of dye is postero-lateral. Figure 14 demonstrates the findings at operation, showing the torn retinaculum with the peroneal tendons retracted out of their normal groove. Treatment of this condition is of course surgical repair of the torn retinaculum and plaster casting. Chronic tears are treated by the method of Jones (30).

In the chronic ankle sprain, usually with a previous history of recurrent inversion sprains, the arthrogram shows a large redundant synovium and formation of pseudo capsule extending beyond the normal anatomical configurations of the ankle joint (Fig. 15). Communications between the ankle joint, various tendon sheaths, and even the subtalar joint will be seen on some arthrograms. No references to such can be found in any of the standard anatomical tests (14, 26, 33). These communications no doubt result from torn tissues at the time of injury. If the clinical picture warrants surgery, we have used the technique of Evans (18) for reconstruction of a lateral ligament. The technique of Watson-Jones (40) results, in our opinion, in prolonged convalescence, and is technically much more difficult.

DISCUSSION

We feel that the arthrogram has clarified the clinical picture considerably in diagnosing the severity of the ligamentous injury. It is a simple out-patient procedure, and its use is recommended for the severe ankle sprain where a tear of the lateral structures is suspected clinically. Its use should be determined by the apparent severity of the lesion on clinical examination. There are numerous

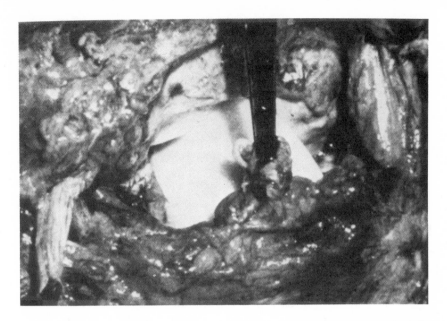

Fig. 11. Type III tear. C.F. ligament in hemostat to left side; A.T.F. to right (talus subluxated and in equinus).

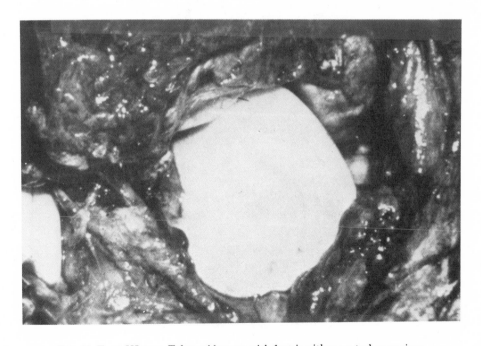

Fig. 12. Type III tear. Talus subluxates with foot in either neutral or equinus.

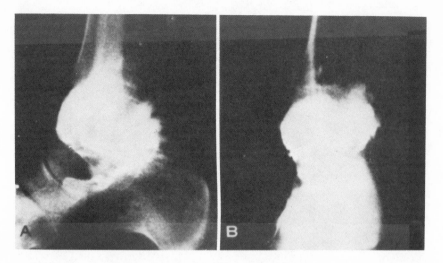

Fig. 13. Acute tear of superior peroneal retinaculum. A. Lateral arthrogram. B. A.P. arthrogram.

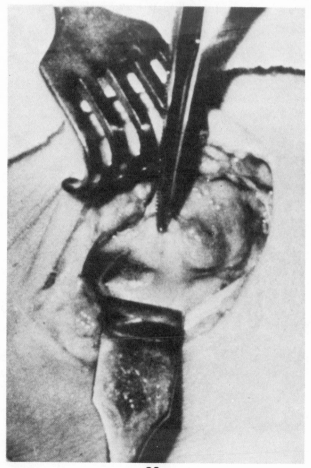

Fig. 14. Operative picture. Torn peroneal retinaculum in hemostat, peroneal tendons retracted below.

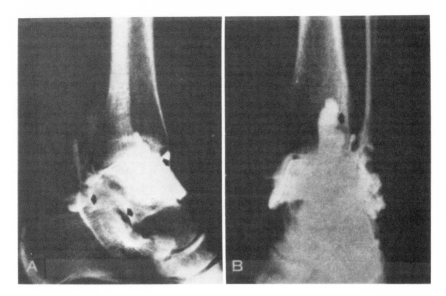

FIG. 15. Chronic recurrent sprained ankle. A. Lateral arthrogram. B. A.P. arthrogram.

references to the use of arthrograms in the literature (3, 6, 7, 19, 25, 27, 42), but few of the authors have correlated their radiological findings with clinical or anatomical interpretation of the pathology presented. Arthrograms are also extremely helpful in defining tears of the deltoid ligament and distal tibio-fibular diastasis.

The method of measurement of severity of the lesion by the use of time-honored talar tilt films is, we believe, grossly unreliable. For the reasons mentioned, many false positives and negatives are encountered by this method. With the use of an arthrogram such false interpretations are excluded.

We feel that a large number of ankle sprains are overtreated, by immobilization for long periods in a plaster cast which is unnecessary in the first place. On the other hand, a substantial number of ankle sprains are more severe than suspected clinically, and so are inadequately treated. The poor results of the overtreated ankle are not too severe, the economic loss and prolonged rehabilitation being the main factors. However, the bad results of the inadequately treated ligament tear may lead to the following symptoms:

1. Recurrent inversion sprains
2. Feeling of insecurity in the ankle
3. Persistent recurrent swelling of the ankle
4. Persistent pain
5. General stiffness and discomfort
6. Local tenderness around the lateral malleolus
7. Dislocating peroneal tendons

It is quite probable that, with recognition and appropriate treatment of the severely "sprained" ankle, such complications can be excluded.

21

SUMMARY

In summary, the authors admit that the impressions drawn from this preliminary report are clinical only, based on radiological and surgical investigation. A review of the literature has been carried out, and this combined with our clinical studies has led us to the following impressions:

1. The use of the term "sprained ankle" is misleading. Severe ligamentous tears and capsular damage may result from a simple inversion injury.

2. The contrast dye arthrography in the ankle may prove to be a valuable adjunct to the diagnosis of severity in the ankle injury and its subsequent treatment.

3. The treatment of this lesion should be based on the severity of the soft tissue damage.

REFERENCES

1. Anderson, K. J., and J. F. Lecocq. 1954. Operative treatment of injury to the fibular collateral ligament of the ankle. J. Bone Joint Surg. *36A:* 825–832.
2. Anderson, K. J., J. F. LeCocq, and M. L. Clayton. 1962. Athletic injury to the fibular collateral ligament of the ankle. Clin. Orthop. *23:* 147–160.
3. Berridge, F. R., J. G. Bonnin. 1944. The radiographic examination of the ankle joint including arthrography. Surg. Gynec. Obstet. *79:* 383–389.
4. Bonnin, J. G. 1944. Hypermobile ankle. Proc. Roy. Soc. Med. *37:* 282.
5. Bonnin, J. G. 1965. Injury to the ligaments of the ankle (Editorial). J. Bone Joint Surg. *47B:* 609–611.
6. Brostrom, L. 1964. Sprained ankles. I. Acta Chir. Scand. *128:* 483–495.
7. Brostrom, L., S. O. Liljedahl, and N. Lindvall. 1965. Sprained ankles. II. Arthographic diagnosis of recent ligament ruptures. Acta Chir. Scand. *129:* 485–499.
8. Charnley, J. 1950. Sprains and dislocations. Practitioner *164:* 314–319.
9. Clark, B. L., A. C. Derby, and G. R. I. Power. 1965. Injuries to the lateral ligament of the ankle: conservative vs. operative repair. Canad. J. Surg. *8:* 358–363.
10. Clayton, M. L., A. W. Trott, and R. Ulin. 1951. Recurrent subluxation of the ankle. J. Bone Joint Surg. *33A:* 502–504.
11. Clayton, M. L., and G. J. Wier, Jr. 1959. Experimental data on the healing of ruptured ligaments. J. Bone Joint Surg. *41A:* 1350.
12. Coltart, W. D. 1957. Sprained ankle. Brit. Med. Assoc. J. *57:* 957.
13. Cotton, R. L. 1961. Soft tissue injuries to the lower extremity. Proc. Nat. Conf. Med. Aspects Sports *3:* 31. A.M.A., Chicago.
14. Cunningham, D. J. Text-book of anatomy. 1947. 8th ed. Oxford University Press, London.
15. De Vries, H. L. 1965. Surgery of the foot. 2nd ed. C. V. Mosby Co., St. Louis.
16. Dziob, J. M. 1956. Ligamentous injuries about the ankle joint. Amer. J. Surg. *91:* 692–698.
17. Elmslie, R. C. 1934. Recurrent subluxation of the ankle-joint. Ann. Surg. *100:* 364–367.
18. Evans, D. L. 1953. Recurrent instability of the ankle: a method of surgical treatment. Proc. Roy. Soc. Med. *46:* 343–344.
19. Freeman, M. A. R. 1965. Treatment of ruptures of the lateral ligament of the ankle. J. Bone Joint Surg. *47B:* 661–668.
20. Freeman, M. A. R. 1965. Instability of the foot after injuries to the lateral ligament of the ankle. J. Bone Joint Surg. *47B:* 669–677.
21. Freeman, M. A. R., M. R. E. Dean, and I. W. F. Hanham. 1965. The etiology and prevention of functional instability of the foot. J. Bone Joint Surg. *47B:* 678–685.
22. Freeman, M. A. R. 1967. Instability of the foot following ligament injuries at the ankle. Proc. Roy. Soc. Med. *60:* 532–534.

23. Freeman, M. A. R., and B. Wyke. 1967. Articular reflexes at the ankle joint. Brit. J. Surg. *54:* 990–1001.
24. Freeman, M. A. R., and B. Wyke. 1967. The innervation of the ankle joint. Acta Anat. *68:* 321–333.
25. Glastrup, H. 1965. Arthrographies in acute ankle injuries. Radiographica *12:* 281.
26. Gray, Henry. 1958. Anatomy of the human body, 32nd ed. Longmans, Green & Co., New York.
27. Hansson, C. J. 1941. Arthrographic studies on the ankle joint. Acta Radiol. *22:* 281–287.
28. Hughes, J. R. 1942. Sprains and subluxations of the ankle joint. Proc. Roy. Soc. Med. *35:* 765.
29. Hughes, J. R. 1949. Radiological diagnosis of recent lesions of the lateral ligament of the ankle. J. Bone Joint Surg. *31B:* 478.
30. Jones, E. 1932. Operative treatment of chronic dislocation of peroneal tendons. J. Bone Joint Surg. *14:* 574–576.
31. Kelley, J. H., and J. M. Janes. 1956. The chronic subluxating ankle. Arch. Surg. *72:* 618–621.
32. Kelly, R. P. 1952. Ankle injuries. J. Kentucky Med. Assoc. *50:* 281–288.
33. Last, R. J. 1959. Anatomy, regional and applied. J. and A. Churchill Ltd., London.
34. Leonard, M. H. 1949. Injuries of the lateral ligaments of the ankle. J. Bone Joint Surg. *31A:* 373–377.
35. Neer, C. S. 1953. Injuries of ankle joint: evaluation. Conn. Med. J. *17:* 580–583.
36. Pennal, G. F. 1943. Subluxation of the ankle. Canad. Med. Assoc. J. *49:* 92–95.
37. Ruth, C. J. 1961. The surgical treatment of injuries of the fibular collateral ligaments of the ankle. J. Bone Joint Surg. *43A:* 229–239.
38. St.-Jacques, R., and C. A. Laurin. 1965. Normal variation of talar tilt of the ankle in children. Canad. Med. Assoc. J. *93:* 695–699.
39. Sherrod, H. H., and J. D. Phillips. 1961. The surgical care of severe sprains of the ankle. South. Med. J. *54:* 1379–1382.
40. Watson-Jones, R. 1955. Fractures and joint injuries, 4th ed. E. & S. Livingstone Ltd., Edinburgh.
41. West, F. E. 1962. Athletic injuries about the ankle and foot. Proc. Nat. Conf. Med. Aspects Sports *4:* 35 A.M.A., Chicago.
42. Wolff, A. 1940. Arthrografi av ankelledd. Nord. Med. *8:* 2449–2456.

DISCUSSION

Dr. Sawnie R. Gaston (New York, New York): I rise for two reasons, first to congratulate Dr. Percy and Dr. Callaghan for a very thorough investigation and excellent presentation. I was fascinated by these anatomic studies, and the authors deserve credit for correlating their studies with the pathologic lesion at operation.

I also rise to emphasize the importance of recognizing more than a sprain in a so-called sprained ankle. These ligament injuries can be very disabling if they are not corrected. Diagnosis depends first on a high index of suspicion, and therefore, when the ankle is swollen beyond your clinical experience of sprained ankle, I think you should suspect that something more has taken place.

You should also consider the clinical picture of swelling: where it is located, whether medial or lateral, and whether the tenderness is over the medial or lateral ligaments or over the lower anterior ligaments.

I have a category of ligament injuries of the ankle that I would like to show you through the use of some slides.

As you can see, these injuries have been induced by various means, and most of them involve external rotation of the foot on the vertical axis of the tibia. We believe that these should be opened, reduced, and bolted.

DR. JOSEPH E. MILLER (Montreal, Quebec): Before commenting on Dr. Percy's paper, I would like to tell you that he has had considerable experience in caring for athletes. Some of you may have heard of one of our local hockey teams, the Montreal "Canadiens." In dealing with professional athletes, one must design treatment with two aims. The first is that the athlete should be helped to recover from his injury as quickly as possible, since time is of the essence. The second is that he should return to competitive sport with little or no remaining disability.

The study just presented by Dr. Percy was stimulated by his seeing a number of patients who required many months to recover from a so-called simple "sprain," or who continued to have minor but disabling symptoms year after year.

The use of arthrography, in effect, differentiates the truly minor injury from the ankle sprain with extensive soft tissue damage. At the risk of repeating some of Dr. Percy's points, I would like to say that arthrography is simple for the radiologist, almost pain-free for the patient, takes only a few minutes, and to date has been free of complications. It also seems clearly to define the state of the ankle.

Dr. Percy's paper is devoted to the question of diagnosis and not to surgical treatment. I am certain we will hear from him again after he has compared the results of his patients treated by operation with those who were treated conservatively. He does, however, suggest tentatively that operation has its advantages in the disrupted ankle. I will say this: I have seen him operate on a few patients, and I am impressed. One cannot help but be surprised in the operating room to see the skin incision made and suddenly observe the entire ankle joint exposed through widely rent capsule and ligaments, so much so that it is in fact easily dislocatable. It is only common sense to think that this kind of injury will recover more completely and more quickly if the ruptured structures are returned to their correct anatomical position and reapproximated by suture.

I believe that Dr. Percy, in his paper, has established that arthrography of the ankle is an important tool to be used routinely, and I forecast that he will, at some future meeting, present evidence to show us when surgical treatment of the severely "sprained ankle" is indicated.

DR. E. C. PERCY (closing): In closing, I would like to thank both Dr. Miller and Dr. Gaston for their discussions.

We have also done work in connection with people injured while on skis. We are well aware of this type of injury, and have used Dr. Gaston's procedure on occasion to help with the diagnosis.

Again, it is much easier to do this technique than to subject the patient to tilt or rotation X-rays. It is far less painful to the patient.

Knee Injuries
in the Adolescent Athlete

Robert L. Larson, M.D.

THE adolescent athlete is not as prone to knee injury as the high school and college athlete. In the three major contact and collision sports—football, baseball, and basketball—23% of the athletic injuries occurred to the knee in those 14 years of age and under, whereas 35% involved the knee in the 15 to 18-year-old age group. In all athletic endeavors in the age group of 14 years and under, 19% of the injuries involve the knee.

Our athletic injury file collected over the past ten years by four orthopedists totals 1,858 athletic injuries; 487 occurred in children 15 years of age and under—26% (Chart I). In this age group, 126 individuals had injuries to the knee (Chart II): sprains accounted for 31%; tears of the meniscii provided 20% of the injuries, two-thirds of which were in the 14 and 15 year olds; 10% were due to tears of the ligaments; contusions, dislocations of the patella; bursitis; epiphyseal separations and Osgood-Schlatter's disease; tendon strains; fractures; and osteochondritis dissecans made up the remainder.

As the child grows and his sports participation becomes more vigorous, the incidence of knee injury increases. In the 126 knee injuries in 15 and under age group, 8 occurred in those of age 8, 9, and 10 years; 35 occurred in the 11, 12, and 13 year olds, and 83 in the 14 and 15 year olds—31 in those 14 years of age and 52 in the 15 year olds (Figure 1).

In the diagnosis of injuries occurring to the adolescent knee, one must be cognizant of conditions which are seen only in children. The epiphyses are the first consideration. Two types of epiphyses are present: traction epiphyses, or apophyses, do not contribute to bone growth but act as insertions for major muscles. The tibial tubercle which is the insertion of the patellar tendon on the tibia is such an epiphysis. The second type is the pressure epiphysis which is found at the end of long bones and contributes to bone growth. The ligaments and fibrous capsule surrounding joints are two to five times stronger to twisting and shearing forces than the epiphyseal cartilage plate. Thus a vector of force transmitted to a knee may result in an epiphyseal displacement. Of the major pressure epiphyses around the knee, the distal femoral epiphysis is the one most commonly involved. This can be explained anatomically by the fact that the medial and lateral collateral ligaments of the knee attach to this epiphysis proximally, whereas their distal attachment to the tibia is distal to the proximal tibial epiphysis. Though sprains and tears to the ligaments are more common, it is important in the adolescent that roentgenograms be made to exclude epiphyseal injury. This is particularly

26

CHART I

ATHLETIC INJURIES
15 YEARS AND UNDER AGE GROUP

Sport	Total No. of Injuries	No. of Knee Injuries	%
Football	128	38	30
P. E.	68	25	37
Skiing	51	17	33
Basketball	51	15	29
Track	47	10	21
Baseball	31	9	29
Others	111	12	11
Total	487	126	26

CHART II

ATHLETIC INJURIES
15 YEARS AND UNDER AGE GROUP

126 Knee Injuries	No. of Injuries	%
Sprains	41	31
Meniscal Tears	27	20
Ligament Tears	13	10
Patellar Subluxation or Dislocation	11	8
Fractures or Epiphyseal Separations	9	7
Contusions and Lacerations	8	6
Bursitis	7	5
Osgood-Schlatter's and Traumatic Tibial Tubercle Epiphysitis	6	5
Tendon Strains	5	4
Osteochrondritis Dissecans	3	2
Internal Derangement (only diagnosis)	3	2
	133*	100%

*Discrepancy due to fact that some injuries to knee contained elements of more than one diagnosis.

so when instability of the joint is detected and a ligament tear suspected. A case in our series illustrates this. A 14-year-old football player sustained a blow to the lateral side of his knee. Gross medial instability was clinically evident on testing. No stress valgus roentgenograms were made prior to surgery for repair of the

Age - 15 years and Under

126 Injuries to the Knee

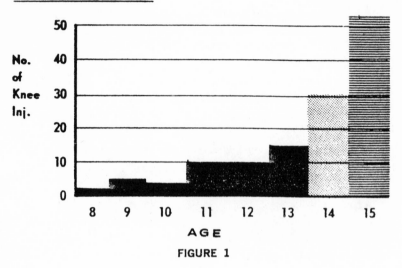

FIGURE 1

"ruptured medial ligaments." At surgery the medial ligaments were intact and the instability demonstrated was due to separation of the medial aspect of the distal femoral epiphyseal plate.

Another injury affecting an epiphysis of the knee is separation of the tibial tubercle. As mentioned, it is at this traction epiphysis that the distal insertion of the quadriceps muscle— the patellar tendon—attaches. Separation occurs as a result of an overload of the isometrically contacting quadriceps as one is decelerating from a jump or coming to a stop from running. In such an action the tibia acts as a lever arm pulling the quadriceps tendon, the patella, and the patellar tendon around the femoral condyles with the mechanical advantage of a rope being wound around the drum of a winch as the knee flexes with foot strike. Since the epiphyseal cartilage plate is weaker than the muscle tendon unit, if something must give due to this dynamic overload, separation at the epiphyseal plate occurs. This "deceleration injury" may cause—(1) partial or complete avulsion of the tongue-like anterior tibial tubercle; (2) partial avulsion of the anterior one-third of the upper tibial epiphyses; or (3) complete separation of the anterior one-third of the upper tibial epiphysis. Such an injury must be suspected in the 12 to 15-year-old who experiences sudden and severe pain after landing from a jump—as in coming down from a rebound in basketball or following a pole vault, high jump, or broad jump.

These separations may occur in a lesser degree of severity from repeated strains to this tendon insertion. In such an instance, the young athlete may start complaining of discomfort over this area after participating vigorously in such an activity as basketball or running. In such a situation, x-rays may reveal slight separation or possibly fragmentation of the tibial tubercle. This, in my opinion, is a traumatically induced epiphysitis.

Osgood-Schlatter's disease is a vascular disturbance causing an ischemic necrosis of the epiphysis of the tibial tubercle. Though its cause is unknown, trauma is the most suspect. The onset of discomfort is usually gradual and not related to any particular accident or injury. There is tenderness and often swelling over the tibial tubercle. Because the etiology of Osgood-Schlatter's disease is still in doubt, insurance coverage is often denied an athlete given this diagnosis. The diagnosis is often used indiscriminately for any discomfort around the tibial tubercle.

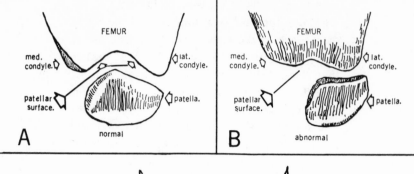

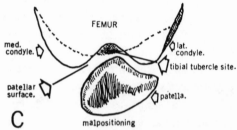

FIGURE 2 A. Normal appearance of patella on modified Hughston view (see Figure 4).
B. Shallow patella-femoral groove with subluxation of the patella laterally.
C. Abnormal patellar development with malposition.

It is important, I feel, to reserve such a diagnosis for those situations where no evidence of trauma to the knee exists—either single or repeated and where roentgenograms reveal a definite necrosis. This condition is often bilateral.

A third condition occurring at the tibial tubercle area which must be considered in the differential diagnosis is a bursitis. Several bursae are located in this area: the prepatellar bursa lying between the anterior surface of the patella and the skin; the deep infrapatellar bursa lying deep to the patellar tendon; and the superficial infrapatellar bursa lying between the tibial tubercle and the skin. The tenderness in prepatellar bursitis and infrapatellar bursitis is elicited proximal to the tibial tubercle. Swelling in prepatellar bursitis is over the patella and in superficial infrapatellar bursitis slightly proximal to the tibial tubercle although this may be difficult to ascertain. In bursitis of the deep infrapatellar tendon, swelling is less readily detected. Roentgenograms will not reveal any abnormality of the tibial epiphysis as in separation or in Osgood-Schlatter's disease.

Patellar dislocation and subluxation are more likely to be encountered in the younger athlete than his older counterpart. Congenital and structural abnormalities of the patella begin to manifest themselves as athletic endeavors are attempted (Figure 2). The contour of the patella can best be judged using the normal sunrise view of the patella (Figure 3A) and the Hughston view (Figure 3B), which gives a better definition of the femoral groove and patellar outline (Figure 4). Where conditions are present which cause an abnormal entry of the patella into the femoral groove such as a deficient patellar groove, a dysplastic patella, or a high riding patella—patella alta (Figure 5), the individual may avoid athletics because of the patellar instability. In this situation, the dislocation is more likely to occur at the beginning of the foot strike to mid-stance as the patella is entering the patellar groove with the controlled elongation of the quadriceps as knee flexion proceeds.

When such patellar abnormalities are less severe or when other defects are present, subluxation and dislocation may become apparent only under the extremes of muscular effort found in athletics. A knock-kneed individual with more lateral insertions of the patellar tendon than normal, a weakened vastus medialis either developmental or from previous injury, and abnormal external rotation of the tibia on the femur are some of the conditions in addition to those mentioned above which predispose to lateral patellar deviation. In these indi-

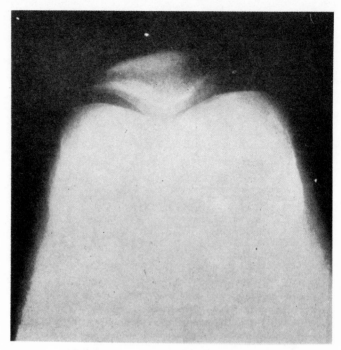

FIGURE 3A Appearance of patella on a "sunrise" view.

viduals, dislocation is most likely to occur during mid-support and take-off when the quadriceps muscle exerts its greatest pull as its extensor explosion occurs. Further enhancement to dislocation occurs with a sudden change of direction from the supporting foot while cutting. This action provides maximum valgus stress as well as external rotation of the tibia on the femur. Thus the requirements for patellar dislocation are present, i.e., maximum valgus of the knee, a position of flexion, and strong quadriceps muscle contraction. If ligamentous relaxation, as often seen in the adolescent athlete, allows increased external rotation of the tibia, or if a direct valgus thrust to the knee by an opposing player is added, patellar dislocation is even more likely to occur.

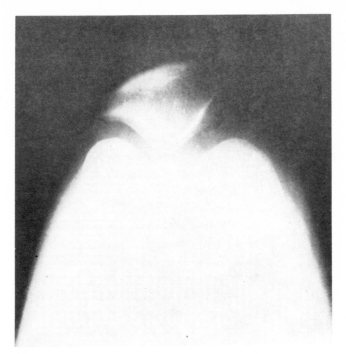

FIGURE 3B Appearance of patella on a modified Hughston view. (This is a roentgenogram of drawing in Figure 2C.)

Often a spontaneous reduction will occur as the knee is straightened. The athlete will give a history of the knee "going out of joint." Clinical examination will reveal tenderness along the medial border of the patella and occasionally a palpable defect where the vastus medialis and extensor retinaculum have been torn away. The athlete will resist efforts to move the patella laterally. If the capsule is intact, joint swelling may be present or if the capsule has been torn the swelling will be more diffuse.

Recurrent dislocation may occur after such injuries with even less muscular exertion due to stretching of the medial retinaculum and resultant loss of its normal action—as a guy wire—to prevent lateral migration of the pa-

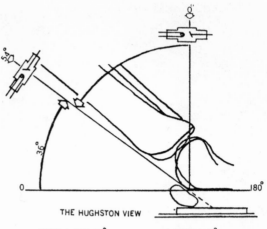

THE HUGHSTON VIEW

TUBE ANGLE 54° — LEG ANGLE 36°

FIGURE 4 Radiographic technique of taking a modified Hughston view. Patient is prone on the x-ray table with the x-ray tube at the 54 degree angle as shown.

BLUMENSAAT'S LINE

(upper part of intercondylar fossa)

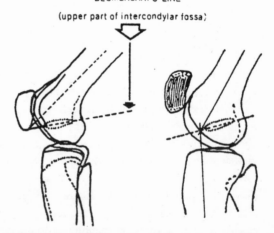

FIGURE 5 Blumensaat's Line—a line projected through the intercondylar fossa on the lateral view with the knee flexed 30 degrees. Normally the distal portion of the patella touches this line. In a high riding patella, the patella sits above this line. (This is not an absolute diagnostic sign since positioning of the knee can vary the position of the patella.)

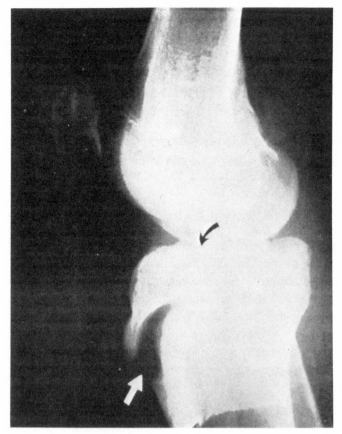

FIGURE 6 Separation of tibial tubercle (white arrow) with fracture through proximal tibial epiphysis and upward angulation (black arrow).

tella. This may be due to a developmental relaxation of these structures.

Treatment of Injuries Peculiar to the Adolescent Athlete

When major epiphyseal separation occurs around the knee, popliteal artery continuity must first be assured. Anterior displacement of the distal femoral epiphysis endangers the artery either by compression or severance. Anterior displacement of the distal femoral epiphysis is reduced by traction on the tibia with

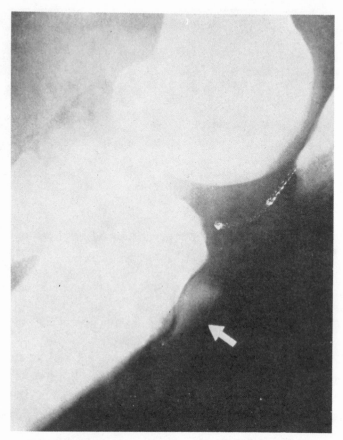

FIGURE 7 Old tibial tubercle epiphysitis with residual bony fragments.

the knee in 45 degrees of flexion. As the knee is further flexed to 90 degrees with traction being maintained, an assistant applies downward firm pressure on the patella. This is accomplished with the leg hanging over the end of the table with a support beneath the junction of the middle and distal one-third of the femur. No pressure should be allowed in the popliteal space because of danger of injury to the popliteal vessels. Displacement may reoccur unless flexion of the knee is maintained to splint the epiphysis by the tightened patellar ligament. Close and continued evaluation of

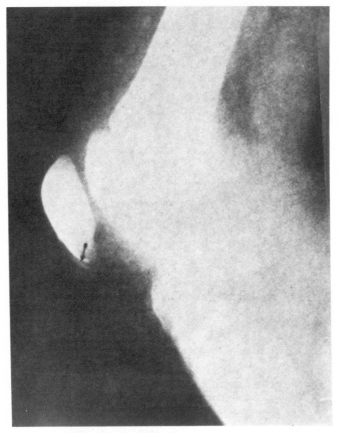

FIGURE 8 Sprain-fracture of lateral superior portion of patellar tendon (Occurred in 10 year old boy running sprints in a relay race.)

circulation in the distal extremity is necessary as swelling may compromise popliteal flow. A spica cast will be necessary to maintain reduction. The knee can be extended 10 to 20 degrees after two weeks.

Posterior displacement of the distal femoral epiphysis is reduced by starting with the knee in 45 degrees flexion and extending the knee with traction. As this is done, downward pressure is applied to the lower one-third of the

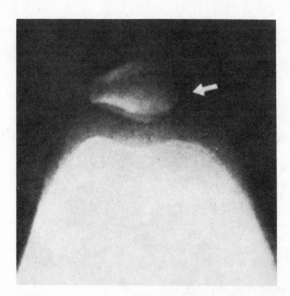

FIGURE 9 Osteochondral fracture from medial patellar facet sustained in basketball when cutting to the opposite side. (The fragment has been retouched for visibility in reproduction.) At surgery, there was a large cartilaginous loose body with a defect in the medial patellar facet.

femur. Since the distal femoral epiphysis has the intact collateral ligaments attached to it as well as the cruciate ligaments, it will retain its relationship to the tibia as this is moved. Immobilization in extension will cause the gastrocnemius heads to tighten and thus splint the epiphysis.

Medial or lateral epiphyseal separations are usually reduced by longitudinal traction and appropriate lateral pressure. Thirty degrees flexion of the knee will relax the tibiocollateral ligament during manipulation.

In our series only one distal femoral epiphyseal displacement occurred. This was the case previously mentioned.

Treatment of separation of the tibial tubercle due to a deceleration injury depends upon the degree of displacement. In the cases of minimal

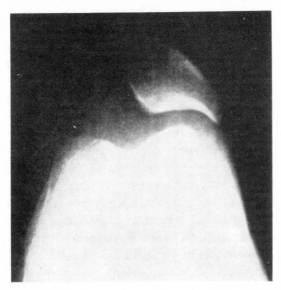

FIGURE 10 Chronic subluxation of patella due to developmental abnormality of patella.

separation, the fractured fragment is molded into position and immobilized in extension by a plaster cylinder until healing takes place. In marked separation, reattachment by suturing or by screw fixation is necessary with cast immobilization until healing occurs which generally takes six weeks.

If, in addition to the separation of the tibial tubercle, a fracture through the anterior one-third of the proximal tibial epiphysis has occurred (Figure 6), accurate reduction is essential to prevent a permanent block to complete extension of the knee. Open reduction, internal fixation, and immobilization is necessary.

Complete separation of the proximal tibial epiphysis is a rare athletic injury but has been reported. When it occurs, prompt assessment of popliteal artery integrity is mandatory.

The treatment of Osgood-Schlatter's disease is generally by rest and restriction of vigorous athletic participation until symptoms subside.

Occasionally, a cylinder cast for complete immobilization is necessary. O'Donoghue has recommended early removal of sequestrated fragments as a means of more prompt and complete recovery.

In epiphysitis involving the entire epiphysis of the tibial tubercle, drilling to re-establish vascularity is recommended by O'Donoghue. Great care must be taken not to disturb the epiphyseal plate of the proximal tibial epiphysis less growth disturbance be induced. In the chronic case where a bony fragment remains separated and a reactive inflammatory process has developed (Figure 7), removal of the loose bony fragments through a split patellar tendon approach is recommended. In an old case where the epiphysis has fused and a bony prominence of the tibial tubercle persists, removal of the bony excrescence may be done if symptoms warrant.

Following immobilization after any of the above forms of treatment, quadriceps exercises with particular emphasis on strengthening of the vastus medialis is required. This will insure quadriceps tension to be spread throughout the extensor expansion rather than being concentrated through the patellar tendon.

Occasionally a sprain-fracture of the attachment of the patellar tendon to the distal patella is seen in the adolescent athlete (Figure 8). This may follow repeated minor traction injuries or a single major strain. Immobilization in a plaster cylinder for six to ten weeks will usually allow bony healing.

When patellar dislocation produces an osteochondral fracture of the medial patellar facet (Figure 9) or lateral femoral condyle, an early surgical approach is indicated with excision or repair of the osteochondral fracture. An acute complete dislocation can be treated by immobilization in a plaster cylinder for six weeks, however, surgical repair to correct the basic developmental defect is usually eventually necessary.

Certainly, if recurrent dislocation, or chronic subluxation of the patella exists (Figure 10), surgical correction is indicated to prevent arthritic changes from developing. The surgery done depends on the basic defect. Medial transplantation of the patellar tendon attachment to the tibia, reefing of the medial retinaculum, construction of a medial band to the quadriceps tendon to provide medial stability, or partial resection of the patella are some of the procedures done to correct these defects.

Tears of the ligaments of the knee or of the meniscii are treated with an early surgical approach as they are in the older athlete.

Conclusions

The adolescent athlete's knee is not the prime target area for injury as it is in the older athlete. This is due in large measure to the lessened forces of contact present in the younger individual. In examining the adolescent athlete after injury, one should keep in mind those injuries peculiar to this age group. Even though the sprained knee is by far the most common knee injury seen (31%), the adolescent athlete with such a primary diagnosis must be carefully evaluated for a possible epiphyseal injury.

References

1. Hughston, J. C.: Recurrent Subluxation and Dislocation of the Patella, Thesis, American Orthopedic Association, 1962. Unpublished.

41

2. Hughston, J. C., and Stone, M. M.: Recurring Dislocations of the Patella in Athletes, So. Med. J., 57:6, p. 623-628, June, 1964.

3. Larson, R. L.: Epiphyseal Injury in the Adolescent Athlete. To be published.

4. Nicholson, J. T.: Epiphyseal Fractures About the Knee, Instructional Course Lectures, Am. Acad. of Orth. Surg., XVIII, 74-83, 1961.

5. O'Donoghue, D. H.: Treatment of Injuries to Athletes, p. 520-522, Philadelphia, W. B. Saunders Co., 1962.

6. Slocum, D. B., and Larson, R. L.: Indirect Injuries to the Extensor Mechanism of the Knee in Athletes, Am. J. of Orth., 6:11-12, p. 248-259, Nov.-Dec., 1964.

The Cross-Body Block, the Major Cause of Knee Injuries

Thomas R. Peterson, MD

Despite the interest in football-incurred knee injuries in recent years, there has been little done to identify and correct the features of the game most likely to cause such injuries.[1-3] Claims of injury reduction with use of artificial turf (Survey of Football and Ankle Injuries, Monsanto Co., 1968) and multiple-shoe variations are not supported by sufficient evidence or controlled study, although such factors may prove, in time, to be important in prevention of injury. A critical appraisal of head and neck injuries by Schneider et al[1] was one of the few realistic studies of game problems which has borne fruit in terms of rule changes, equipment modifications, and attention to certain hazardous blocking and tackling methods.

A similar study at the University of Michigan was directed to the appraisal of knee injuries, the major disability problem in football. The work completed in the early phase of this study clearly indicates that the maneuver known as the cross-body block causes more knee injuries than all other factors combined.

The material studied consisted of all available records from the athletic departments and hospitals of the University of Michigan and Michigan State University and also from the Detroit Lions professional team and from local high schools. The communication concerns derangements of the knee joint including fractures of the condyles of the tibia and the femur and dislocations of the patella. The review series included only those cases in which the documentation was sufficient, the pathologic changes well-defined, and the disability significant. The mechanism of trauma was specifically identified through interview with team physician or trainer, review of game films, or interview with the injured, player. In cases investigated since the study began in 1966, the documentation has been more complete and the cases reviewed have been consecutive for the teams mentioned and for all high school

Table.—Total Injuries Studied Prior to 1967*

Game Maneuver	No. of Injuries	% of Total Injuries
Cross-body block	103	54
No contact	42	22
Tackled	22	12
Blocked	4	2
Pileup	18	10
Total	189	100

*The cross-body block causes more knee injuries than all other mechanisms combined.

team injuries treated at St. Joseph Mercy Hospital, Ann Arbor, Mich.

For the 15-year period prior to 1967, a total of 189 cases of knee injury were reviewed. The Table shows the number of injuries which resulted from each of the game maneuvers which are listed as the major subdivisions of the Table. In the separation of these causes, cross-body block is listed as a specific blocking technique, and the category "blocked" includes all other blocking methods used in offensive play. "Tackled" refers to the traditional procedure for stopping a runner, and "pileup" designates the group of injuries in which there was multiple-player contact and a single mechanism could not be incriminated. It is recognized that the force factors in knee injuries are often the same whether they occur in tackling, blocking, or in the entanglement of the pileup. put in own word

If one football-playing technique is associated with a disproportionately high number of injuries, it must be concluded that the injurious forces are an inherent part of that technique. The proportions in the Table clearly implicate the cross-body block as the major cause of knee injury in football with 54% of the 189 cases associated with this specific

1. Classical cross-body block and fixation of defender's foot demonstrated in professional football photo.

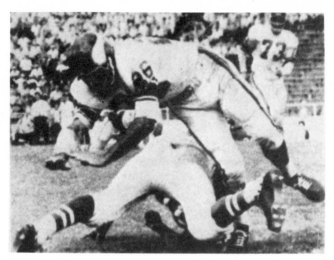

technique. The 1967 and 1968 seasons were surveyed separately to allow comparison of the injury rates during these years with those of the earlier period. Fifty-two percent of 36 knee injuries studied in 1967 and 53% of 34 knee injuries studied in 1968 were caused by the cross-body block. These cases bring the total injuries studied to 259 with 54% caused by the same blocking method. The consistency of the injury pattern in the periods surveyed is impressive. Although the number of injuries varies from year to year on the different teams, there is a persistent dominance of this one mechanism in causation.

Correlation of Mechanism and Pathologic Findings

Although knee injuries do occur without external contact, the results of this study confirm Stewart's finding[5] that the large majority are the result of stress applied from the outside. As shown in the Table, 22% of the knee injuries in this series occurred in the absence of contact between players. Analysis of the pathologic changes in these cases of no-contact injury showed a definitely higher incidence of cartilage tears than was noted in contact injuries, supporting the impression that such damage often occurs through torsional stresses alone. Where the injuries resulted from external contact forces, the most common result was ligament disruption. Comparison of injuries at different levels of skill and physical maturity showed that the cross-body block causes more knee injuries at the high school and college level than among the professional players. This probably reflects a more sophisticated approach related to experience with injuries and more subtle blocking methods in the professional game.

2. Cross-body block is comparable to the thrust of a railroad tie against the unsupported knee.

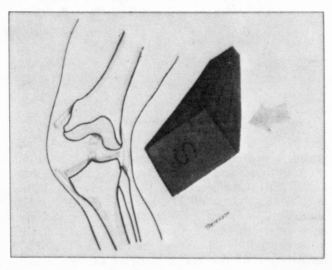

The Cross-Body Block
If any single game technique or blocking method

46

is to be indicted as a major cause of injury, it should be examined in the light of its use on the football field and its importance to the game. Analysis of the destructive forces involved in the cross-body block requires an understanding of the specific motions and the intensity of the physical forces employed in this blocking method.

The cross-body block is one of the offensive blocking techniques used to prevent the defensive player from interfering with the forward progress of the football. The blocker throws himself horizontally at the opponent's knees in an attempt to upset him (Fig 1). The "roll block" is the follow-through part of this technique and is also the secondary effort in upright blocking methods when the initial thrust is missed. Here, the blocker rolls his body into the opponent horizontally, like a rolling log, in a continuing effort to catch the defender's legs. A whipping motion of the blocker's legs is the final attempt to delay the opponent when the primary means fails.

The cross-body block is used chiefly in the open field where considerable momentum can be developed. It is one of the more dramatic and exciting moments in the game when a defender is cut down or upended, and it usually occurs when the player is unaware of the impending block. This means that the block is coming from the side rather than from the front, and under these circumstances the maneuver is termed "blind-siding." The "crack-back block" is a specialized form of blind-siding used by flanking men who come back into the scrimmage area and attempt to strike linebackers while they are oblivious to the blocker's approach. The illegal block termed "clipping" refers to any blocking effort directed at the opponent from behind. From the standpoint of sportsmanship, there seems to be little distinction between the illegal act of clipping and the legal cross-body block which catches the defender unaware.

In recent years, the cross-body block has been used increasingly as a substitute for traditional tackling procedures. This is seen most frequently when a runner is forced out of bounds and when a pass receiver is cut down by a defensive halfback. In open field play, in this day of larger and faster players, the cross-body block can be likened to the thrust of a railroad tie against the side of the unprotected knee (Fig 2). Coaches have recognized

47

3. Blocker's unprotected flank is vulnerable in cross-body block.

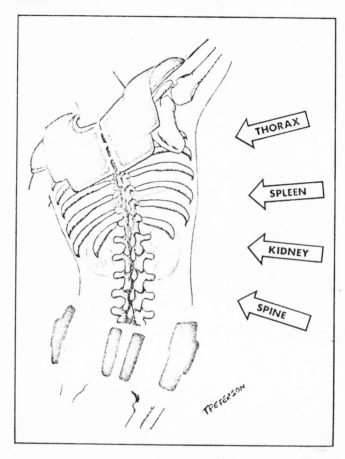

both the dangers and the undeniable effectiveness of this technique by designating special players—"suicide squads"—for the open field play during kickoffs and punt returns. Football coaches and officials have recognized the dangers, but have never specifically identified the cross-body block as the true cause of the injuries they have noted.

Injury to the Blocker

Injury to the blocker who uses the cross-body block has not been described. In fact, injuries sustained by the blocker are likely to be of a more serious nature than those to the player who is blocked. The classical technique in delivering the cross-body block exposes the unprotected ribs and flank with obvious hazard to the lungs and abdominal viscera (Fig 3). The standard hip and shoulder pads offer no protection at all for the thorax and flank when the body is stretched out in this position. This study identified cases of rib fractures, forearm fracture, pneumothorax, splenic rupture and contusion, and lumbar transverse process fracture incurred by the cross-body blocker. The total number of these injuries is small relative to the knee injuries recorded, and this is surprising when the absence of protection for the blocker's flank is considered.

The final whipping effort of the blocker's leg was responsible for two complete knee ligament ruptures to blockers in this survey. As in cervical spine and head injuries, which are related to certain blocking and tackling techniques, the possibility of serious trauma to the cross-body blocker must be weighed in the consideration of the value of this particular blocking method.

Rule Changes Related to Knee Injuries

Historically, the Football Rules Committee has attempted to reduce the incidence of game injuries. In 1922, effort was made to eliminate clipping by ruling that it was illegal "to throw the body from behind across the legs (below the knees) of a player not carrying the ball." The rule was not to apply to play in the scrimmage area. Thus the hazard of the cross-body block was recognized at that time, but it was seen as dangerous only when it came from behind. Since that time, the term "clipping" has been applied to any block from behind, but injury has been rare when the blow was delivered above the knees. Injuries from the cross-body block, however, have continued at the same or increasing levels of frequency.

In 1967, the rules committee, alarmed by the incidence of injury due to the crack-back block declared in rule 9 that "an offensive player who is outside this area (scrimmage zone) and in motion toward the ball when it is snapped is not permitted to clip in this area." Again, the basic problem was not corrected and the crack-back block has continued to disable linebackers because most of these injuries are due to the cross-body block with clipping hardly a factor.

Football officials have been obliged to approve a block delivered from the side while penalizing the same block delivered from behind when injury may result in both cases. From this it is concluded that a blow from the side when the defendent can not see his assailant is proper and sportsman-like. It is my opinion that elimination of the cross-body block would obviate all concern about clipping.

Recommendations

Haddon[6], in surveying research problems in sports as related to health, made the following recommendations:

Where potentially injurious amounts of mechanical forces are employed, as in boxing and football, their timing, magnitude, and direction must be quantitatively considered in relation to the injury threshholds of the target tissues and organs. Special attention should be given to the study of sport modifications or substitutions that would reduce or eliminate hazardous forces to the brain, spinal cord, or other vital structures.

The ultimate damage to the knee joints after major knee injuries with and without surgical treatment is well-recognized by those familiar with articular degeneration and joint trauma.[7-9]

If the cross-body block can be responsible for approximately 50% of all serious knee injuries as well as being hazardous to the blocker, it is reasonable to evaluate the specific role of this game maneuver and to consider alteration of the rules. Although opinion is divided among coaches, many feel that the aims of cross-body block can be accomplished by other means and do not teach this method. At the early high school level, however, the cross-body block is taught routinely and it becomes an instinctive maneuver for most football players particularly in desperation efforts. Effective legislation will be necessary as the means of prompt control and the impetus to reeducation.

As a result of this study, I believe that football rules should be changed to eliminate the cross-body block. If other factors such as artificial turf and shoe variations should decrease the total number of knee injuries, there is reason to believe that the same percentage related to the cross-body block will persist.

More specific recommendations as to the type of rule changes are not the province of this communication. It is recognized that elimination of the cross-body block would cause a major change in football methods and tradition, but the possibility of a significant reduction in the number of serious knee injuries as well as minimization of the potential for visceral injury must be seriously considered by football's rules-makers.

James Feurig, MD, and the Athletic Department of Michigan State University; Kent Falb and the Detroit Lions Football Co.; and James Hunt, Lindsy McLean, and Lenwood Paddock and the University of Michigan Athletic Department assisted in this investigation.

References

1. Hawk, K.G.: "Football Injury Survey," in *Procedings of the 31st Annual Meeting, American Football Coaches Association,* 1954, pp 41-47.

2. Quigley, T.B.: Injuries to the Ligaments of the Knee, *Clin Orthop* 3:20-28. 1954.

3. O'Donoghue, D.H.: Surgical Treatment of Fresh Injuries to the Major Ligaments of the Knee, *J Bone Joint Surg* 32-A:721-738 (Oct) 1950.

4. Schneider, R.C., et al: Serious and Fatal Football Injuries Involving the Head and Spinal Cord. *JAMA* 177:362-367 (Aug 12) 1961.

5. Stewart, M.J.: *Management of Ruptures of Cruciate and Collateral Ligaments of the Knee,* Instructional Course Lectures, American Academy of Orthopaedic Surgeons, 1968-1969.

6. Haddon. W., Jr.: Principles in Research on the Effects of Sports on Health, *JAMA* 197:885-888 (Sept 12) 1966.

7. Fairbank, T.J.: Knee Joint Changes After Meniscectomy. *J Bone Joint Surg* 30-B:664-670 (Nov) 1948.

8. Du Toit, G.T.: "Internal Derangements of the Knee," in *Instructional Course Lectures.* American Academy of Orthopaedic Surgeons, 12:9-34, 1955.

9. Ghormley, R.K.: Late Joint Changes as a Result of Internal Derangements of the Knee. *Amer J Surg* 76:496-501 (Nov) 1948.

Varsity Football

Knee and Ankle Injury

MURLE LAURENS ROWE, M.D.

Football injuries of the knee and ankle have been a major area of concern to all connected with the game. Local, state, and national statistics on football injuries are in general agreement that 1 boy in 3 who plays high school football will sustain an injury requiring medical care, causing lost time from participation each season. Of these injuries, 1 in 3 will involve the knee or the ankle.

O. W. Hanley, and others have called attention to the number of knee injuries, in particular, which occur without contact when the player cuts or pivots on a foot firmly fixed to the turf by a conventionally cleated football shoe. Various technics have been suggested to "de-cleat" the shoe in the hope that by reducing the fixation of foot to turf, torsional stresses could be dissipated before damage was done to the ankle or knee in much the same fashion as does the safety release ski binding.

One technic for partial decleating is to replace the two heel cleats of the conventional football shoe with an ordinary street shoe heel or, more conveniently, with a specially made plastic disk. Another is to use short, soccer-type cleats, stubby rubber

Presented at the Second Annual Symposium on the Medical Aspects of Sports, February 8, 1969, sponsored by the Medical Society of the State of New York.

TABLE I. Types of shoes and cleats

Type of Shoe and Cleat	Number
HC (high shoe, conventional heel cleats)	349
HD (high shoe, disk heel, conventional sole cleat)	190
LC (low shoe, conventional heel cleat)	278
LD (low shoe, disk heel, conventional sole cleat)	379
SE (soccer or rubber cleats)	129
Total	1,325

cleats, or ripple soles in place of the conventional long, conical, football cleat. Preliminary reports indicate that the mini-cleat, which is used on the synthetic rug types of playing surfaces, cuts the incidence of knee and ankle injuries.

During the 1967 football season a State-wide study of New York State high school football players using various shoe and cleat combinations indicated some diminution in the severity of knee and ankle injuries among players using the disk heel on a low-cut shoe, but design defects in the study prevented solid conclusions and the study, with minor modifications, was repeated during the 1968 season.

A separate, somewhat more detailed study of the same problem has been conducted in an 11-county area designated Section Five of the New York State Public High School Athletic Association, under the sponsorship of Mr. Lewis C. Obourn, president of the New York State Public High School Athletic Association and with the assistance of Mr. Roger Bunce, football chairman of Section Five.

Section Five study

Section Five lists 80 schools which play high school football at the varsity level in 11 leagues. All 80 schools were invited to participate in the study. Data were collected by the coaches of the varsity squads

on special study forms. Information concerning school grade, position played, hours
of practice and of game participation, shoe
and cleat type worn, and history of previous knee or ankle injury was recorded for
every squad member. Additional data
including date and circumstance of injury,
diagnosis, time lost from participation, and
any additional pertinent comments were
recorded for boys sustaining knee and ankle
injuries. No attempt was made to control
the type of shoe or cleat used except that
presentations at regular annual athletic
injury conferences in the area had stressed
the importance of knee and ankle injuries
and the possibility that these injuries could
be reduced by decleating.

Completed study forms were returned by
the coaches or athletic directors of 44
schools. Detailed information was received on 1,325 high school varsity football
players. Table I shows the types of shoes
and cleats worn by the study group.

With the exception of the group designated SE (special equipment) which included a variety of stubby cleat types on
both high and low shoes, all equipment
groups comprised a sufficient number of
players to allow significant experience to be
recorded. The SE group was carried
through the calculations for whatever
indications might be derived as to the effect
of further decleating.

The entire study group of 1,325 sustained 100 knee injuries (7.5 per cent of
participants) and 77 ankle injuries (5.8 per
cent of participants). These incidence
percentages are well in line with state and
national statistics of past years and would
indicate a generally acceptable level of
reporting.

Incidence of knee and ankle injuries in
terms of percentage of participants for
each of the five equipment groups is shown
in Table II. More striking than the outstandingly good record of any equipment
group is the rather outstandingly bad
performance of the LC (low shoe, conventional cleat) group.

54

TABLE II. Five equipment group (per cent)

Injuries	Total Group	HC	HD	LC	LD	SE
Knee	7.5	7.2	7.4	10.4	6.6	5.4
Ankle	5.8	4.6	5.8	8.3	5.8	3.9

TABLE III. Injuries per 100,000 hours of participation

Site	Total Group	HC	HD	LC	LD	SE
Knee	68	64	66	96	58	47
Ankle	52	41	52	77	51	34

Incidence of injury

With further analysis of data, it became clear that variables other than the type of shoe and kind of cleat worn were involved in the incidence of knee and ankle injuries. Most significant of these were game participation versus practice participation and exposure of backfield men as contrasted with linemen. To evaluate these and other variables it became necessary to express the incidence of knee and ankle injuries as rate per participation time rather than as a simple percentage of participants. For convenience in numbers, this rate was established as the number of injuries per 100,000 hours of participation. Table III shows the conversion of knee and ankle injury incidence to this rate for each equipment group. The information conveyed is the same as in the percentage-of-participants injury incidence (Table II), in which it appeared that the highest incidence of injury occurred in the group using the low-cut shoe with the conventional long conical cleats (LC).

Using the same method of calculation, the injury rate was determined for practice, participation, and game-participation hours. Since the ratio between knee and ankle injuries was approximately the same for all equipment groups, knee and ankle injuries were lumped together for this calculation. For the total group, the rate of knee and ankle injury was 69 per 100,000 practice hours and 657 per 100,000 game hours of participation. In other words, the risk of knee or ankle injury is approximately ten times as great in game exposure as in practice participation. Approximately the same ten-fold increased risk in game versus practice was found in all equipment groups.

It was also found that there was a significant difference in the amount of game exposure between equipment groups. Expressed in terms of percentage of total participation hours spent in games, the differences are shown in Table IV.

TABLE IV. Game exposure (per cent)

Total Group	HC	HD	LC	LD	SE
8.6	7.5	7.9	9.3	9.8	8.1

TABLE V. Injury rate adjusted for game exposure

Rate	Total Group	HC	HD	LC	LD	SE
Combined knee and ankle	120	105	118	173	109	81
Adjusted for game exposure	120	111	122	166	103	83

Since the risk of injury is so much higher in games than in practice, and since there is a significant difference in the amount of game exposure of the various equipment groups, it was necessary to correct the injury incidence rate for each equipment group to adjust for its degree of game exposure. This was done mathematically for the combined knee and ankle injury incidence rate. Table V shows the unadjusted combined knee and ankle injury rate for each group and, in the line below, the rate adjusted for the degree of game exposure.

Significant differences in injury rate now appear, particularly when the low-cut shoe with the conventional cleat (LC) is compared with the low-cut shoe with the disk heel (LD), the two equipment groups showing the highest percentage of game exposure.

Using the same rate method, the relative risk of backs and linemen were compared for the group as a whole and for each equipment group. For the total group, the rate of knee and ankle injury in backfield men was 178 per 100,000 hours of participation. For linemen, the rate was 86 per 100,000 participation hours. There was no significant variation from this ratio in any of the separate equipment groups. In other words, the risk of knee or ankle injury is approximately twice as great for a back as for a lineman.

It was found that there was a significant

TABLE VI. Exposure of backfield men (per cent)

Total Group	HC	HD	LC	LD	SE
37	15	33	40	56	37

difference in the number of hours of backfield man exposure as compared with lineman exposure in the various equipment groups. Expressed in terms of percentage of total participation hours contributed by backfield men, the differences are shown in Table VI.

Since the risk of injury is twice as great in backs as in linemen, and since there is a significant difference in the hours of backfield man exposure between the various equipment groups, it was necessary further to adjust the injury incidence rate for each equipment group. Table VII shows the unadjusted rate for each group, the rate adjusted for game exposure as in Table V, and, finally, the rate adjusted for backfield man exposure.

Equipment combinations

It appears that of the widely used equipment combinations, the low-cut shoe with the disk heel significantly reduces the incidence of knee and ankle injuries, especially when compared with the low-cut shoe, conventionally cleated, which is the second most widely used shoe-cleat combination for backfield men. The low rate in the special equipment group, where further decleating was carried out, tends to support the principle that reduction of fixation of foot to turf will prevent knee and ankle injuries, although the numbers of players using the special equipment were too small to be highly significant.

For full meaning of the rate differences for the various equipment groups, the figures must be translated back into numbers of injuries to participants at the individual team level. On the average, each football team puts in about 3,300 hours of

TABLE VII. Adjusted injury rates

Rate	Total Group	HC	HD	LC	LD	SE
Crude knee and ankle	120	105	118	173	109	81
Adjustment for game exposure	120	111	122	166	103	83
Adjustment for backfield participation	120	132	126	162	90	83

participation per season. Therefore, the total participation of 30 teams would equal 100,000 hours. If the difference in injury rate between the low-cut shoe with the disk heel (LD) and the low-cut shoe with the regulation cleat (LC), which is 72 knee and ankle injuries per 100,000 hours, is divided among 30 teams, then each team would

TABLE VIII. Severity of injury

Lost Days	HC	HD	LD	LD	SE
Knee (100)					
0–7	11	4	11	8	3
8–14	5	4	10	2	1
15–30	1	1	2	5	2
31 plus	8	5	6	10	1
Ankle (77)					
0–7	11	7	14	11	3
8–14	1	3	3	7	1
15–30	0	0	3	4	0
31 plus	4	1	3	0	1

avoid about 2 knee and ankle injuries per season if they used low-cut, disk heel shoes instead of low-cut conventionally cleated shoes. The low-cut, disk heel shoe will, on the average, prevent 1 knee or ankle injury per season if used in preference to a high-cut shoe for each team.

No conclusions could be drawn from this study as to the effect of any shoe-cleat combination in minimizing the severity of knee and ankle injuries. Factors other than the severity of injury influenced the number of days lost from participation which was the measuring stick for severity. It was felt that medical review of the injured would be necessary to establish meaningful data concerning severity. Table VIII shows the severity of knee and ankle injuries in terms of days lost from participation for each equipment group.

Further study of the injured developed interesting but not surprising or controversial findings. These are shown in Table IX.

Conclusions

A numerically limited but somewhat

concentrated study of 1,325 varsity football players in Section V of the New York State Public High School Athletic Association would indicate that the low-cut shoe with the disk heel is the safest shoe-cleat equip-

TABLE IX. Study of injured players (177)
(knees and ankles)

Considerations	Number of Injuries
Positions	
Back, offense	52
End, offense	6
Line, offense	22
Back, defense	43
End, defense	11
Line, defense	43
Dates of injuries	
August	2
September 1 to 14	32
September 15 to 30	53
October 1 to 15	46
October 16 to 31	26
November	18
Game vs. practice	
Game	84
Practice	93
Activity when injured	
Tackling	23
Being tackled	52
Blocking	15
Being blocked	60
Pileup	13
No contact	14

ment combination in common use today. Use of this equipment combination would, on the average, save each team 2 knee and ankle injuries per season over the most dangerous equipment combination, the low-cut shoe with conventional cleats, and 1 knee or ankle injury per season over other commonly used equipment combinations.

The small experience (129 players) with soccer style or rubber cleats indicates this may be an even better equipment selection than the low-cut, disk heel shoe. On the basis of the indications from this study, it would appear that a low-cut shoe with a disk heel and soccer or stubby, rubber sole

61

cleats might be the best selection of all from the standpoint of the prevention of knee and ankle injuries.

REHABILITATION OF INJURED FOOTBALL PLAYERS[1]

A. B. CORRIGAN, M.B., B.S., M.R.A.C.P., M.R.C.P. (Edin.), M.R.C.P.
D.Phys.Med.

OVER the last ten years, there has been a great change
in the management of sporting injuries, with increasing
emphasis on active methods of rehabilitation in contrast
to previous techniques of prolonged immobilization
(Ferguson, 1965; Corrigan, 1965). It is generally agreed
that the régime to follow is (i) emergency treatment,
followed by (ii) early and intensive physiotherapy. For
the emergency treatment, Trickett (1965) uses the
mnemonic "ICE"—"I" for ice, "C" for compression, "E"
for elevation of the affected part. This is continued over
the first 24 hours of the injury.

After this, physiotherapy is commenced in a supervised
programme that is gradually increased. The techniques
used are those used ideally in rehabilitation medicine.
We are dealing not just with an injury, but with an
injury in a particular individual who is to return to
a particular place in a particular team or event. Thus,
the programme can be compared to the concept of total
care for the individual's illness that characterizes the
approach of modern-day physical medicine specialists.

The physiotherapy techniques used in soft-tissue injuries
consist basically of the application of heat (by shortwave diathermy or ultra-sonics) and exercises. The
injured part is exercised within the limits of pain
tolerance; exercise begins gradually, and the *tempo* is
gradually increased. It is obvious that there needs to
be adequate supervision of the exercise programme by a
physiotherapist. The aim is gradually to increase strength
and extensibility of the affected part. At the same time,
the other areas of the body that are not injured are
exercised, either by specifically designed exercises or in a
general activity type for programmes—as, for example,
games. It is for these reasons that special athletes' clinics
have been built, for example, at Lewisham Hospital and
Sydney Hospital.

---

[1] Those taking part in this trial included Dr. W. Buckingham,
Dr. N. Caldwell, Dr. W. J. Cook and Dr. M. Henry.

One of the factors that limits this programme is the presence of pain and swelling. Indeed, pain is an almost universal complaint, and yet it is quite uncommon for adequate analgesics to be prescribed. If this active therapy is to be undertaken, then relief of pain is of prime importance.

During the 1965 Rugby League season, a survey was carried out on injuries; 97 cases were recorded, all being sufficiently severe to warrant medical attention. It was not intended that the incidence of injuries in the number of players at risk be assessed, but only that the type of injuries that occur be recorded. There has been no similar survey of Rugby in Australia, though Ferguson made a survey of Australian Rules football injuries.

At the same time, an attempt was made to relieve pain and swelling by the use of oxyphenbutazone ("Tanderil", Geigy). For purpose of standardization of treatment and of analysis of results, it was used for five days, starting immediately after the injury was received. Placebo treatment was not given, because the injuries were all relatively severe and the players were unwilling to use placebo tablets; hence, this is a form of consecutive care therapeutic evaluation.

AIMS OF INVESTIGATION

The aims of the investigation were: (i) to analyse the the types of injury occurring during a Rugby League season and to grade them according to severity; (ii) to observe the overall result of therapy by estimating the time of return to full function; (iii) to observe whether analgesia is an aid to rehabilitation and if there are any side effects.

DETAILS OF THE INVESTIGATION

The types of injuries and their degree of severity are shown in Table 1. This shows that the most frequent injuries are joint sprains and muscle injuries. These

TABLE 1

Type of Injury	Degree			
	Total	Mild	Moderate	Severe
Indirect muscle injury	13	3	8	2
Direct muscle injury	10	0	8	2
Joint sprain	35	1	28	6
Bone injury	11	3	5	3
Bursitis	14	1	11	2
Tenosynovitis and tendinitis ..	7	0	7	0
Painful subcutaneous contusions	6	1	4	1
Total	97	9	72	16

were then graded into degrees of severity; for example,

ligament injuries in joint sprains may be graded as follows: (i) minimal, in which there are only a few fibres torn; (ii) severe, in which almost all fibres are torn and invariably a hæmarthrosis is present; (iii) moderate, which comprise most of the cases and are intermediate between the previous two categories. Muscle injuries are classified into two types: (i) indirect injuries or muscle pulls in which muscle fibres are torn; (ii) direct injuries as a result of a direct blow resulting in muscle hæmatoma.

Bone injuries may be either a subperiosteal hæmatoma, classified as a mild or moderate injury, or a fracture, classified as a severe injury. There were three fractures in this series, one of a thumb metacarpal and the other two of a terminal phalanx, an injury that causes little disability to footballers.

Bursitis may occur either as the result of a direct injury or else from overuse in training. The subcutaneous contusions were all of the shins—an occupational hazard of footballers.

RESPONSE TO TREATMENT

The response of these injuries to treatment was assessed by noting the response of pain and swelling to therapy. This was classified as follows: (i) excellent—full recovery; (ii) good—recovery sufficient to allow training; (iii) fair—relief of symptoms, but not sufficient to allow training; (iv) poor—no appreciable difference in symptoms.

The patients were all treated for five days, and then were assessed on the following day. Results are shown in Table 2. Two had side effects of the tablets, and treatment was discontinued. Seventeen patients had only a fair or poor response to treatment, and so had to have a major modification of their régime and hence were not followed up any further for the purposes of this paper.

Those patients who did not show any improvement at all are listed in Table 3. They do not reveal any particular injury which consistently fails to respond to this régime.

TABLE 2
Response of Pain and Swelling to Treatment

Severity of Injury	Response[1]			
	Excellent	Good	Fair	Poor
Mild	7	1	1	0
Moderate	37	21	6	7
Severe	7	5	2	1
Total	51	27	9	8
	78		17	

[1] Treatment discontinued, two cases.

The remaining 78 who were improving at this sixth-day assessment, were then followed up until fully recovered.

Those injuries originally classified as mild took an average of six days, moderate injuries took an average of eight days, and severe injuries took an average of 15 days, for return of full function. During this time, physiotherapy and tablets were continued, as indicated.

TABLE 3

Poor Results

Subject's Number	Age (Years)	Nature of Injury	Severity of Injury
1	26	Epicondylitis	Moderate
2	20	Sprain, left ankle	Moderate
3	20	Sprain, right ankle	Moderate
4	25	Injury to cervical part of spine	Moderate
5	23	Fracture, right first metacarpal	Severe
6	32	Trochanteric bursitis	Moderate
7	27	Left olecranon bursitis	Moderate
8	25	Thoracic intervertebral disc lesion	Moderate

SIDE EFFECTS OF TREATMENT

There were two patients who could not tolerate the tablets, one because of gastric irritation and one because of urticaria. Therapy was discontinued in both cases.

COMMENTS

This paper is concerned with the treatment of injuries to highly-trained athletes, who were seen immediately after injury and received intensive and early therapy. It is not suggested that similar results would occur in people of sedentary habits or with injuries treated after a time lapse.

Ferguson (1965) states that prolonged immobilization of patients with football injuries is no longer necessary, and writes: "It is in the field of soft tissue injury that the most spectacular advances have been made in treatment." The relief of pain is of prime importance if this more active therapy is to be undertaken, as pain prevents movement. Analgesics should be used for this, as other possible tablets, such as muscle relaxants or enzymes given by mouth, do not have any true analgesic properties.

The analgesic action of "Tanderil" is well documented. It is a break-down product of butazolidine, and so the two drugs are similar in their actions (Cardoe, 1959; Hart, 1959). This pronounced analgesic effect is due to an anti-inflammatory effect, as the drug has no central analgesic effect (Husted, 1962).

The ideal dosage to be used was a problem; because of the short-term nature of these injuries, relatively high dosages can be given. Fitch (1965) used 600 to 800 mg. per day for five days. Paul (1965), in treating injuries in American grid-iron players, used 600 to 800 mg. on the first day and tapered the dosage off to 200 mg. on the fifth day. In this trial we used 600 mg. per day for two days, and then 400 mg. per day for the next three days. As was indicated previously, this dosage can be continued if indicated.

The response of pain and swelling in 78 of the cases

was considered to be either good or excellent, and so allowed of fuller use of physiotherapy services. We believe that since pain is usually what brings these patients to see a doctor, adequate analgesia should be ensured by the doctor.

SUMMARY

Ninety-seven cases of football injury are reviewed from the point of view of type of injury, response to therapy and time of the player's return to full function. The results are presented.

ACKNOWLEDGEMENTS

Thanks are offered to those doctors of football clubs who cooperated in recording the players under their care, and to Dr. N. Percy, of Geigy (A/sia) Pty. Ltd., for his generous supply of "Tanderil" tablets.

REFERENCES

CARDOE, N. (1959), "Controlled Trial of G.27202 in Rheumatoid Arthritis", *Ann. rheum. Dis.*, 18 : 244.

CORRIGAN, B. (1965), "Treatment of Muscle Injuries in Sportsmen", *MED. J. AUST.*, 1 : 926.

FITCH, K. (1965), "Muscle Injuries", *Sports Med. J.*, 1 : 40.

FERGUSON, A. S. (1965), "Injuries in Australian Rules Football", *Ann. gen. Pract.*, 10 : 155.

HART, F. D. (1959), "Phenylbutazone and its Derivatives", *Brit. med. J.*, 1 : 1087.

HUSTED, E. (1962), "The Effect of G.27202 (Tanderil, Geigy) on Post-operative Discomfort", *Acta odont. scand.*, 20, No. 3.

PAUL, J. (1965), "Documenta Geigy: Preliminary Report of XI International Congress of Rheumatology, Argentina, December".

TRICKETT, P. C. (1965), "Athletic Injuries", Meredith, New York.

Tennis Leg

Avrum I. Froimson, MD

Tennis leg is a painful condition of partial tearing of the medial belly of the gastrocnemius, caused by over-stretching the muscle by concomitant ankle dorsiflexion and full knee extension. Contributory factors are muscle fatigue and degenerative changes. Simple conservative treatment is effective and permanent disability does not result. Prodromic calf aching has been discussed and permits preventive measures to be taken. A diagnosis of plantaris tendon rupture is erroneous.

THE RECENT increase in popularity of tennis in this country makes necessary better understanding by physicians of certain injuries peculiar to the sport. Although much has been written about "tennis elbow," little has been written about "tennis leg." An acutely painful calf injury with typical symptoms and signs, tennis leg is readily recognized and easily treated. The clinical picture is generally but erroneously attributed[1] by tennis players and physicians alike to tear of the plantaris tendon, but the true nature of the problem is a partial tear of the medial gastrocnemius muscle belly at or near the musculotendinous junction.

Clinical Picture

A tennis player, usually of middle age, while serving the ball or stretching to the side for a difficult shot, feels that something has struck the back of his calf. He may think it is a ball from a neighboring court or something thrown at him. Accompanying this feeling in the calf occasionally is an audible snap, sounding like a twig breaking. Momentarily there is no pain, but as soon as the player takes his next step there is intense pain in the posteromedial part of the calf midway between knee and ankle. The player may collapse or faint. In most cases he has to be helped off the tennis court because of the intense pain in the calf by his attempting to walk.

Physical examination reveals sharply localized tenderness and frequently a palpable defect in the medial muscle belly of gastrocnemius at or above the musculotendinous junction. After a few hours, swelling obscures the palpable defect and it is a few days until the depression in the muscle can again be felt. Plantar flexion power is diminished and there is no muscle tone in the medial head of gastrocnemius for a few weeks. Characteristically, the lateral head of the gastrocnemius and the popliteal space are not tender and the heel cord is intact. After a few days ecchymosis may be seen over the medial calf, extending distally along the heel cord to the ankle. There may be slight ankle edema.

The Prodrome

A previously unmentioned characteristic of this injury is premonitory calf pain a day or two prior to injury. My interest in this injury began when I sustained the injury and recalled that the day before there had been a dull aching in the calf muscle of the affected leg. Subsequently, questioning patients specifically about this point, about half recalled similar prodromic calf discomfort. The significance of the prodrome is discussed later in this communication.

Review of the Literature

To my knowledge, the earliest mention of this problem was in 1884 when Hood[2] described "lawn tennis leg." Arner and Lindholm,[3] in 1958, presented their experience with 20 cases and refuted the theory of plantaris tendon tear by surgically exploring five of their 20 patients, finding in each instance a transverse rupture of the medial gastrocnemius belly at the musculotendinous junction with gaps of 1 or 2 cm. In every patient explored the plantaris muscle and tendon were intact.

They pointed out that anatomically the musculotendinous junction of plantaris was in the lateral popliteal area beneath the lateral gastrocnemius head and therefore distant from the painful medial calf defect. Further, they pointed out that plantar flexion weakness would not be associated with rupture of the insignificant plantaris. To their observations one can add that when the plantaris tendon is stripped and removed to be used for flexor tendon grafting, there is only transitory popliteal tenderness and minimal calf pain without weakness or inability to walk normally.

Mechanism of Injury

A combination of maximum knee extension and ankle dorsiflexion is necessary to produce this lesion. In discussing injuries to the musculotendinous unit, Brewer[4] pointed out the vulnerability of certain muscles to such injury because each such musculotendinous unit activated or crossed two joints. In addition to the triceps surae, which was ruptured in 23% of such injuries in the lower extremities, the particularly vulnerable muscles were biceps femoris, semimembranosus, and rectus femoris, all of which cross two joints. When the knee is fully extended and the ankle fully dorsiflexed the gastrocnemius is stretched to maximum length, increasing the tension on the elastic elements of muscle enough to tear it in certain instances.

Furthermore the gastrocnemius is one of the "muscles of short action." A muscle of short action itself cannot affect the complete range of motion possible in the joints on which it acts, and is therefore subject to overloading. The gastrocnemius muscle, contracting at maximum length, is therefore overloaded.

Added to the mechanical factors of stretching is the phenomenon of failure of relaxation. It has been pointed out that muscle relaxation is an active physiological function and not merely a passive occurrence. Muscle stiffness represents a decline of such physiological elasticity with fatigue. The prodromic symptoms of muscle aching prior to the actual occurrence of tennis leg represents this stiffness of fatigue. Unable to fully relax, a muscle is more liable to rupture.

Other contributory factors have been studied by other authors, McMaster[5] experimentally produced weakness in the musculotendinous unit by impairment of vascular supply. Arner and Lindholm[3] demonstrated abnormal histologic findings in the muscle and tendon in middle-aged patients.

To explain why tennis leg is a phenomenon of the middle-aged tennis player one must consider the factors stretching the gastrocnemius muscle in players of all ages. The flat-heeled tennis shoe allows exaggerated ankle dorsiflexion, which tightens the heel cord, while sudden knee extension increases the tension on the muscle belly from above. Not only does tennis leg not occur in young players with the same stresses, but sometimes it occurs in middle-aged persons not even playing tennis. This condition has been encountered in persons simply stepping down from a curb or step ladder or while slowly running or jogging. The incidence in middle age is understood when one considers in addition the factors of slowed reaction time, muscle stiffness, decreased muscle and tendon blood flow, and possible abnormal histologic findings (structural weakness).

Treatment

Since the diagnosis is based on the classical signs and symptoms, x-ray examination is not necessary. The injured leg should be elevated and ice bags applied to the calf for at least 24 hours, longer if desired. Proteolytic enzymes given orally have seemed to reduce the duration of the acute reaction. No controlled study has been done to prove this. Ideally, the patient should stay off his foot for 24 to 36 hours. During the first day or two he will frequently require crutches for ambulation. After the initial painful interval, ambulation can be facilitated with considerable reduction of pain by elevating the heel of the shoe on the involved side from ¾ to 1 inch. This is simply done by having the cobbler nail an extra heel onto the shoe. This alleviates discomfort by reducing the pull on the injured gastrocnemius and relaxing the calf muscle. Because the built-up shoe makes the limb seem at bit longer, the patient keeps his knee slightly flexed, further relaxing the injured gastrocnemius muscle belly. A cane may be useful. Although elastic support has been recommended by other authors, it has been found to cause increased discomfort. Unless there is undue ankle swelling, no external support is utilized. An elastic stocking gives more comfort than elastic bandaging.

The patient can generally have the extra heel removed within two weeks, but will not be able to walk barefoot comfortably for approximately three or four weeks. Until all calf pain has subsided, he must not attempt to play tennis again, since reinjury is common and prolongs the period of disability. An average of five weeks should have elapsed from the time of injury until his return to the tennis court. During the first few weeks after resumption of play, the heel should be elevated approximately three-eighths of an inch by a felt pad inside the shoe.

The prognosis is excellent. The dimpling in the medial gastrocnemius head persists along with reduction of gastrocnemius tone and strength for many months. Some measurable calf atrophy may be detectable for one year. After complete healing, reinjury of the same leg has not been observed. In several patients the opposite calf has been affected by the same injury later.

Perhaps by recognizing the importance of the prodromic calf pain, this injury can be prevented. Where possible, physicians, tennis professionals, and teachers should instruct players to avoid play if a calf muscle is already painful. Unless there is measurable restriction of ankle dorsiflexion due to heel cord tightness, prophylactic stretching of the normal calf musculature in an attempt to prevent tennis leg is useless.

References

1. McLaughlin, H.L.: *Trauma,* Philadelphia: W.B. Saunders Co., 1959, p 367.
2. Hood, C.: On Lawn-tennis Leg, *Lancet* 1:728, 1884.
3. Arner, O., and Lindholm, À.: What is Tennis Leg? *Acta Chir Scand* 116:73-77 (Dec 8) 1958.
4. Brewer, B.J.: "Mechanism of Injury to the Musculotendinous Unit," in *Instructional Course Lectures,* St. Louis: C.V. Mosby Co., 1960, vol 17, pp 354-358.
5. McMaster, P.E.: Tendon and Muscle Ruptures, *J Bone Joint Surg* 15:705-722, 1933.

72

Treatment of Tennis Elbow with Forearm Support Band

BY AVRUM I. FROIMSON, M.D.

Although the pathological lesion in tennis elbow has not been convincingly demonstrated, it appears that most methods of treatment have in common the reduction of tension in the common extensor origin on the lateral humeral epicondyle. Conservative remedies include rest, cock-up splints, and elbow braces, while surgical methods relieve tension directly by fasciotomy, muscle stripping, or tendon lengthening. To provide a simple method of achieving this desired relief of tension, I have designed a forearm support band that is being produced commercially.

The support is a 5.4-centimeter wide band of heavy-duty non-elastic fabric lined with foam rubber padding to prevent slipping. The band is easily applied with Velcro fasteners encircling the forearm just below the elbow (Fig. 1). Tension is adjusted to a comfortable degree with the muscles relaxed so that maximum contraction of the wrist and finger flexors and extensors is inhibited by the band. The patient is advised to use the support only during actual play to avoid excessive tightness and to remove it during periods of inactivity to avoid venous congestion and edema.

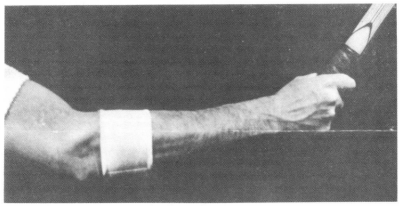

Fig. 1

Tennis player wearing forearm support band showing correct level of application.

In acute cases treatment with the forearm band is augmented with local anesthetic and steroid injections into the tender tissues distal to the lateral epicondyle. Oral phenylbutazone or aspirin may also be prescribed.

Forty patients have been treated with this support. Twenty-three of the twenty-eight who were treated with the forearm band and injection therapy were relieved of pain, while ten of the twelve treated with the forearm band alone were relieved.

Once relieved, patients are advised to continue using the band during play for at least a year to avoid recurrence.

This tennis-elbow support has several advantages. It is very light in weight, easy to apply, and does not interfere with elbow motion thereby allowing normal tennis strokes. One size of support fits all patients for easy dispensing or prescribing. The support is inexpensive.

Tennis Elbow: Diagnosis, Pathology and Treatment

Nine Severe Cases Treated by a New Reconstructive Operation

RICHARD C. GARDNER, M.D.

Tennis elbow is one of the most common lesions of the upper extremity. Its diagnosis is relatively simple, but its pathology and treatment in resistant cases are topics of considerable controversy. It has been my opinion that the reason for this diversity is that no one has ever operated on an acute case of tennis elbow and personally observed the pathology. In the cases previously reported, surgery has only been attempted *late* in those cases resistant to all forms of conservative therapy, and when fibrosis has formed and has masked the original pathology. This paper will show not only the pathology found in 2 cases operated on in the *acute* stage but also will offer a new, more logical reconstructive operation for such resistant cases.

DIAGNOSIS

The diagnosis of tennis elbow is easily made. It usually occurs gradually in those people subject to repeated pronation and supination of the upper extremity, such as dentists, surgeons, secretaries, carpenters, bowlers, golfers or tennis players. In *acute* cases, the usual cause is a sudden extension of the elbow, supination of the forearm with a motion involving tension of the extensor muscles—such as throwing a heavy load or the backhand swing in tennis. Pain is localized just distal to the lateral epicondyle; there is weakness of grasp and pain on supination or pronation of the forearm. The chief complaint is often that the patient cannot lift or play sports without pain in the region of the lateral epicondyle.

The chair test (Fig. 1) is the most important clinical finding. The more severe the tennis elbow, the more positive the test. The patient is asked to lift a chair with one hand, which is pronated. Severe pain in the region of the lateral epicondyle is experienced by all those with a tennis elbow. Unless the test is positive, the defect is not very symptomatic. The stress test (Fig. 2) is another valuable clinical tool. The physician attempts to flex the patient's wrist while the extensor muscles are contracting against the patient's resistance. This will also cause pain in the region of the lateral epicondyle, but I feel this test is not as diagnostic as the chair test. On palpation, the area of maximum tenderness is usually just on, or distal to, the lateral epicondyle, in the region of the conjoined tendon of the extensor muscles. There may be pain on stressing the joint inward with the elbow extended (varus stress).

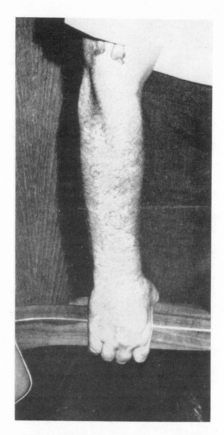

PATHOLOGY IN THE LITERATURE

There are diverse opinions about the true pathology of tennis elbow. Osgood (1922)[8] thought it was due to an inflamed extra-articular bursa beneath the conjoined tendon (radiohumeral bursitis). Trethowan (1929)[10] thought there was a synovial outpocketing of the radiohumeral joint. Cyriax (1936)[3] suggested small tears in the conjoined tendon, and Moore (1952)[7] spoke of

a synovial fringe with evidence of inflammation. Bosworth (1955)[1] identified the pain with the orbicular ligament, and Kaplan (1959)[6] with neuritis of the branches of the radial nerve.

I have had the opportunity to explore 2 elbows acutely and at these times the pathology has been clear.

CASE REPORTS

One patient, a 15-year-old girl, developed a tennis elbow from delivering newspapers by throwing them from her bicycle. After a particularly vigorous throw, with the elbow fully extended, the forearm supinated, and the wrist flexed, she felt a snap in her elbow. She was unable to lift anything thereafter. On examination there was some swelling just distal to the lateral epicondyle. The chair and stress tests were markedly positive. She was treated with rest, local anesthetics and steroids, but continued to have pain for 2 weeks without improvement. On surgical exploration, there was a complete *linear* tear of the conjoined tendon, radial collateral ligament, and capsule of the elbow just distal to the lateral epicondyle (see Fig. 3). A reconstructive operation was done and the result has been excellent with a follow up of more than 17 months.

A 45-year-old female suffered tennis elbow after she lifted a heavy bag while working in a laundry and tried to swing it with the elbow extended, the forearm pronated, and with the extensor muscles under tension. She felt a sudden snap in the elbow region and was unable to lift after this. On examination she had tenderness just distal to the lateral epicondyle

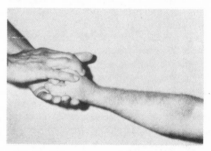

FIG. 2. *The stress test.* The physician tries to flex the wrist against resistance, while the patient contracts his extensor muscles. There is pain experienced near the lateral epicondyle.

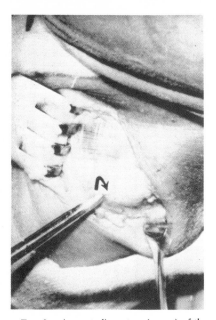

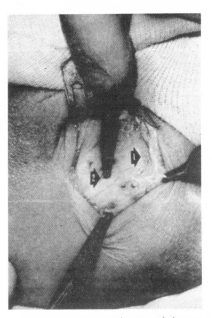

FIG. 3. An acute *linear* tear (arrow) of the conjoined tendon, radial collateral ligament, and capsule of the elbow joint just distal to the lateral epicondyle. Surgery was performed on this 15-year-old girl with a severe tennis elbow, after no improvement in 2 weeks. Original trauma was from throwing a newspaper while on a delivery route.

FIG. 4. An acute *circular* tear of the conjoined tendon, radial collateral ligament, and capsule of the elbow joint (2) just distal to the lateral epicondyle (1) in a 45-year-old female laundry worker. Surgery was performed in this severe case after it did not improve in 2 weeks. Original trauma was from swinging a laundry bag.

and markedly positive chair and stress tests. On surgical exploration, there was a complete *circular* tear of the conjoined tendon, the radial collateral ligament and the capsule of the elbow joint just distal to the lateral epicondyle (see Fig. 4). An operation was done. Excellent results continued a year postoperatively.

The operation performed will be described later.

TREATMENT IN THE LITERATURE

For the majority of patients, conservative treatment of tennis elbow is often successful. This consists of physical therapy, heat and diathermy, or local injections of anesthetic and steroids. There have been a great many procedures recommended for resistant

cases. Cyriax[3] suggested manipulation, while Trethowan[10] and Moore[7] have recommended excision of the synovial fringe of the radiohumeral joint. In 1953, Spencer and Herdon[9] suggested either a fasciotomy or stripping of the common extensor origin in resistant cases. In 1955, Bosworth[1] excised a portion of the orbicular ligament, but in 1965, he suggested a division of the conjoined extensor muscle as well.[2] In 1961, Garden[5] reviewed cases of resistant tennis elbow treated by tenotomy of the extensor carpi radialis brevis, just above the wrist. In 1967 Friedlander[4] reported 9 cases treated by section of the common extensor origin and resection of the orbicular ligament.

Patient	Age–Sex	Occupation	Initiating Trauma	Results
1. C.C.	45–F	Laundry worker	Swinging a laundry bag (Compensation Case—Acute)	Excellent—12 months
2. L.M.	50–M	Clerical	Bowling (Chronic)	Excellent—17 months
3. P.M.	35–F	Housewife	None	Excellent—12 months
4. H.W.	15–F	Newspaper delivery girl	Throwing a newspaper (Acute)	Excellent—17 months
5. B.M.	36–F	Secretary	None	Excellent—19 months
6. L.G.	39–M	Fireman	Bowling (Chronic)	Excellent—18 months
7. B.H.	47–F	Housewife	None	Excellent—18 months
8. T.M.	35–M	Clerical	Bowling (Chronic)	Excellent—12 months
9. L.B.	41–M	Computer operator	Golfing (Chronic)	Excellent—3 months

CLINICAL EXPERIENCE AND METHOD

The author has had extensive clinical experience with more than 100 cases of tennis elbow. All but 9 cases improved with conservative care. In 9 cases undergoing surgery, six had some history of trauma, either acute or chronic. Two of the 6 gave a history of *acute* trauma with severe disability and these cases were operated on acutely. Three cases had no history of trauma. The 9 operative cases are summarized in Table 1. All had a markedly positive chair and stress test and pain localized just distal to or on the lateral epicondyle. The pathology in the acute cases was either a *circular* or *linear* tear in the common extensor tendon, radial collateral ligament, and capsule of the elbow joint. The seven chronic cases all showed fraying of the same elements, indicating repair of the tear by fibrosis. No bursae, synovial outpocketing, or abnormal orbicular ligaments were found in surgery.

ANATOMY

The conjoined common extensor tendon is composed of the tendinous origins of 4 muscles—the extensor carpi radialis brevis, the extensor digitorum communis, the extensor digiti quinti, and the extensor carpi ulnaris.

PATHOLOGY

The tear in acute cases and the fraying in the chronic cases are found just distal to the lateral epicondyle. Contrary to most claims, the lesion may be intra-articular since it may involve not only the common extensor

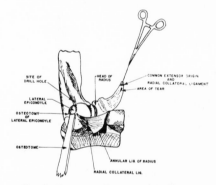

Fig. 5. Reconstructive surgery for tennis elbow. The conjoined tendon, radial collateral ligament (anterior portion) and the capsule are all held in an inverted U-shaped flap. The lateral epicondyle is excised down to cancellous bone with an osteotome. The flap is then reattached through a drill hole ⅜ of an inch proximal to the lateral epicondyle on the humerus. This shortens the extensor apparatus, thereby strengthening it. The tear or fraying is approximated to the raw cancellous area of the excised epicondyle.

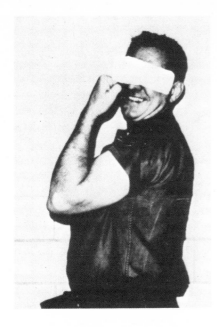

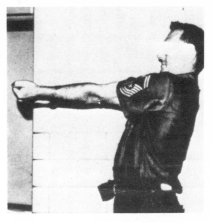

FIGS. 6, 7. Six weeks following the operation, this champion bowler scored the highest average of his career. He demonstrates an excellent full range of motion without pain or loss of strength in grasp or extensor power.

tendon origin, but also the radial collateral ligament and capsule of the elbow joint.

RATIONALE OF THE OPERATION

Fasciotomy, stripping of the common origin of the extensor tendons, or excision of the orbicular ligament may relieve the pain of the tennis elbow, but may also weaken the radial collateral ligament of the joint or dorsiflexion power of the wrist or hand.

Logically, if the pathology is a tear, then this tear must be repaired and the areas stabilized to prevent a recurrence. The operation to be described does just that, and, in addition, is designed to increase the power of dorsiflexion and lateral stability of the elbow joint.

METHOD

The 9 cases charted have all had the same operative procedure. A pneumatic tourniquet is not necessary, but simplifies the operation. General or regional anesthesia may be used. A 6 cm incision begins just above and posteriorly to the lateral epicondyle and swings anteriorly over the common extensor tendon origin. The fascia is incised in the line of the incision. This brings into view the muscle belly of the anconeus, the common extensor origin, and the lateral border of the muscle belly of the mobile wad. Care is taken to protect the radial nerve which lies just under the brachioradialis. The tear in acute cases or the fraying in chronic cases is then sought out. Heavy silk is inserted as a figure 8 into the common extensor origin, deep enough to include the radial collateral ligament and capsule of the elbow joint which is intimately associated. An inverted U-shaped incision is then made in the common extensor tendon origin and including the capsule and the radialcollateral ligament (anterior portion) as well. The incision extends just distal to the head of the radius. (See Fig. 5.) The orbicular ligament is not excised. By means of a periosteal elevator, the lateral epicondyle is delineated and the triceps muscle retracted posteriorly. An osteotome is then used to remove the lateral epicondyle down to cancellous bone. By means of a %4-inch drill bit, a hole is made perpendicular to the bone ⅜ of an inch proximal to the previously removed epicondyle. A large, curved, thin needle is then threaded with the heavy silk and centered through the new hole. The assistant flexes the elbow and dorsiflexes the wrist while the surgeon ties the knot. The object in this shortening procedure is to bring the area of fraying or tear over the raw cancellous bone of the removed epicondyle. Additional 2–0 silk sutures are then placed in the tear itself and the flap sutured to the anconeus muscle laterally and the extensor carpi radialis longus muscle medially. The fascia is then closed along with the subcutaneous tissue. A subcuticular stainless steel wire is then used to suture the skin. No cast, splint, or immobilization is used postoperatively. The patient's arm is placed in a sling and told to move the elbow as soon as the pain subsides. The strong fixation of the tendon to the bone allows early active motion.

RESULTS

All patients were followed for an average of 14.2 months after the operations. All were asymptomatic, had full range of motion in the elbow, and their strength of grasp and dorsiflexion power were excellent. None had pain over the area previously involved and all were satisfied with the result. One patient, a champion bowler, bowled the highest score of his life 6 weeks after the operation. Before the operation he had difficulty competing (Figs. 6, 7).

There were no wound infections. One patient had enough postoperative pain to warrent placing him in a splint for one week, but all patients except one (a compensation case) were back to partial work 2 weeks following surgery.

DISCUSSION

Although small, a certain percentage of patients with tennis elbow will ultimately require surgery.

The author feels that this operation is reconstructive in nature and further strengthens the elbow joint, grasp and extensor power. No excision of the orbicular ligament, operative lengthening with consequent weakening, fasciotomy or stripping of the common extensor tendinous origin are done. It offers early active motion and rehabilitation, as well as early discharge from the hospital and return to work. In retrospect, the name of this common disease entity should really be changed from tennis elbow to "torn elbow." Although common among Davis Cup players, it may be found in those with any occupation demanding repeated pronation and supination motions of the forearm.

SUMMARY

In most of the author's 100 cases of tennis elbow improvement followed conservative therapy. Nine cases came to surgery, including 2 severe cases following acute trauma that showed no improvement after 2 weeks. Pathology in the acute cases was either a circular or linear tear in the common extensor origin, the radial collateral ligament and the capsule of the elbow joint. Seven cases were classified as chronic and the pathology found in surgery was fraying of the same elements.

A new reconstructive operation in the 9 cases has shown excellent results in a follow-up period which averaged 14.2 months. (See Table 1.)

REFERENCES

1. Bosworth, D. M.: The role of the orbicular ligament in tennis elbow, J. Bone Joint Surg. 37A:527, 1955.
2. ———: Surgical treatment of tennis elbow—A follow up study, J. Bone Joint Surg. 47A:1933, 1965.
3. Cyriax, H. H.: Pathology and treatment of tennis elbow, J. Bone Joint Surg. 18: 921, 1936.
4. Friedlander, H. L., Reid, R. L., and Cape, R. F.: Tennis elbow, Clin. Orthop. 51: 109, 1967.
5. Garden, R. S.: Tennis elbow, J. Bone Joint Surg. 43B:100, 1961.
6. Kaplan, E. B.: Treatment of tennis elbow (Epicondylitis) by denervation, J. Bone Joint Surg. 41A:147, 1959.
7. Moore, M., Jr.: Radiohumeral synovitis, Arch. Surg. 64:501, 1952.
8. Osgood, R.: Radiohumeral bursitis, epicondylitis, epicondylalgia (tennis elbow), Arch. Surg. 4:420, 1922.
9. Spencer, G. E., and Henderson, C. H.: Surgical treatment of tennis elbow, J. Bone Joint Surg. 35:A421, 1953.
10. Trethowan, W. H.: Tennis elbow, Brit. Med. J. 2:1218, 1929.

Real Tennis Elbow

D. N. GOLDING.

SIR,—Strain of the common extensor origin at the lateral epicondyle due to lawn tennis is an uncommon cause of tennis elbow, as compared to direct or indirect trauma of an unsporting nature. "Table tennis elbow" and "badminton elbow" are also occasionally seen, but as far as I know the condition has never been described in connexion with real tennis, as in the following case.

A 34-year-old professional real tennis player had recurrent pain in the region of the right elbow, which was severe enough to prohibit him playing in matches. On examination, he had the classical signs of lateral epicondylitis—that is, tenderness over the epicondyle, a positive Mills's sign, and pain on resistant dorsiflexion of the wrist while the elbow was extended. The condition responded satisfactorily to conservative treatment consisting of a hydrocortisone injection into the common extensor origin at the tenoperiosteal junction.

Real tennis, the forerunner of lawn tennis, is played on an enclosed court with a hard ball. The racket is roughly pear-shaped, one side being slightly flattened, giving it a rather asymmetrical appearance. The grip is similar to that used in lawn tennis, and the standard stroke is carried out with a chopping motion, rather like the volley stroke used in lawn tennis. The patient informs me that this necessitates greater strength of wrist and forearm than other court games, and therefore might well predispose to tennis elbow.—
I am, etc.,

Ball Throwers' Fracture of the Humerus

Six Case Reports

MARTIN S. WESELEY, M.D., AND PHILIP A. BARENFELD, M.D.

Fracture of the humeral shaft resulting from indirect trauma has been previously documented. Conwell and Reynolds[3] stated that the shaft of the humerus can be broken by muscular action and that this is the most common site of fracture from this cause. The American Medical Association's handbook on Standard Nomenclature of Athletic Injuries[6] indicated that fracture of the humeral shaft may result from forcible muscular action, such as throwing. Scudder[7] also mentioned that fracture of the middle or distal third of the humeral shaft can occur from muscular action as in throwing a baseball. Callender[2] stated that the humerus is the most common bone fractured by muscular action. He, too, related the injury to the act of throwing and implicated the deltoid

ACKNOWLEDGEMENTS: The authors would like to thank Peter LaMotte, M.D., John H. Muehlstein, M.D., and Mark Pitman, M.D., for contributing their cases to this series.

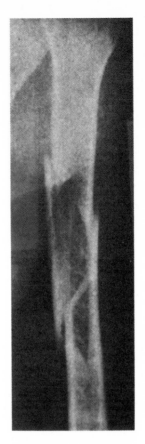

FIG. 1. (Case 1) Acute comminuted fracture, right humeral shaft.

muscle as the culprit. The fractures start just below the deltoid insertion and are supposedly the result of sudden arrest of the bone by the deltoid and the acquired impetus of the lower end of the humerus. O'Donoghue's,[5] McLaughlin's[4] and Watson-Jones'[9] texts made no mention of this type of mechanism.

Six cases of fracture of the humeral shaft resulting from violently throwing a ball are presented in this study. We treated 3 of these cases and 3 were contributed by other orthopaedic surgeons. After reviewing these cases, we analyzed the mechanism of fracture, presenting a somewhat different emphasis

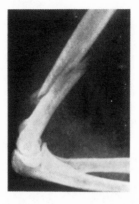

Fig. 2. (Case 2) Early callous formation, spiral oblique fracture, right humeral shaft.

than previous explanations.

CASE REPORTS

Case 1. F.M., a 30-year-old man, was playing right field in a softball game on June 23, 1964. As he threw a ball toward home plate, he felt a sudden sharp pain in his right arm and noted a deformity. He was taken to the emergency room of a local hospital where he was treated by one of us. Roentgenograms revealed a comminuted fracture of the middle third of the shaft of the right humerus with a large medial butterfly fragment (Fig. 1). The patient was treated with a hanging cast and the fracture united uneventfully. Laboratory studies to rule out any pre-existing bone pathology were all within normal limits. This patient rarely participated in athletics.

Case 2. W.B., a 27-year-old man, was playing right field in a softball game on July 20, 1966. He threw a ball toward home plate, felt a sudden sharp pain in his right arm, and could not move it. He was taken to the emergency room of a local hospital where one of us was consulted. Roentgenograms revealed a simple spiral oblique fracture of the junction of the upper and middle thirds of the right humerus. The fracture was treated with a hanging cast and it united uneventfully (Fig. 2). This patient participated in athletics frequently.

Case 3. S.B., a 27-year-old man, was playing in a softball game on June 10, 1964. He threw a ball from the outfield, heard a snap, and felt a sudden sharp pain in his arm. Roentgenograms revealed a comminuted fracture of the upper half of the right humerus (Fig. 3). The fracture

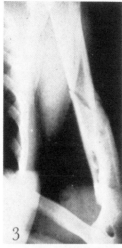

FIG. 3. (Case 3) Acute comminuted fracture, right humeral shaft.

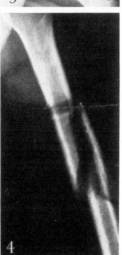

FIG. 4. (Case 4) Acute comminuted fracture, right humeral shaft.

healed uneventfully. This patient had sustained a fracture of the lower half of the same bone 3 months previously which had healed well.

Case 4. R.S., a 21-year-old professional baseball pitcher was throwing a fast ball while warming up on June 5, 1963. He thought he heard a pistol shot as he felt a sudden sharp pain in his right arm. Roentgenograms revealed a comminuted fracture of the middle third of the right humerus with a large lateral butterfly fragment (Fig. 4). He was treated with plaster splints and the fracture healed uneventfully.

Case 5. T.H., a 28-year-old man, was playing shortstop in a softball game on August 18, 1967, when he relayed a throw home from the outfield and felt a snap in his right arm. He stated he had thrown as hard as he could. He was taken to the emergency room of a local hospital where

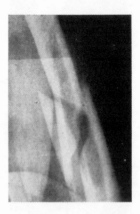

Fig. 5. (Case 5) Acute comminuted fracture, right humeral shaft.

he was treated by one of us. Roentgenograms revealed a comminuted fracture of the middle third of the humerus with two large butterfly fragments (Fig. 5). The patient, at that time, had a partial ulnar nerve palsy. He was treated with a hanging cast and healed uneventfully. The partial ulnar nerve palsy recovered completely. This patient played softball in a league weekly for several years.

Case 6. J.L., a 20-year-old male college student threw a snowball violently and felt his arm snap on the evening of January 22, 1966. Roentgenograms revealed a long spiral oblique fracture of the distal humeral shaft (Fig. 6A). A hanging cast was applied, but the position was unacceptable, and 5 days post-injury an open reduction with screw fixation was performed (Fig. 6B). The screws were subsequently removed in June, 1967. The patient had no complaints, but he subsequently lacked 5 degrees of flexion and extension.

DISCUSSION

In analyzing the mechanics which contribute to the production of this fracture, we feel the emphasis placed on muscular contraction is incorrect. This lesion is produced by a violent torque applied perpendicular

86

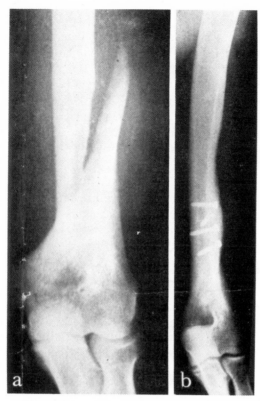

Fig. 6A, B. (Case 6) a, Acute spiral oblique fracture, right humeral shaft. b, postoperative appearance of fracture.

to the shaft of the humerus. There are several forces acting on the humerus during the act of throwing a small, fairly heavy ball. These forces change constantly throughout the act of throwing. Slocum[8] divides the act of throwing into 4 steps: the initial stance, the wind up, the forward action to release, and the follow through. At the start of the third step in throwing, the shoulder is abducted, externally rotated and extended, and at the end of step 4, the shoulder is adducted, internally rotated and flexed. The elbow is flexed to some degree until the very end of the follow-through motion. The powerful muscles about the shoulder contribute considerably to the force of the thrown ball. Both Slocum[8] and Bateman[1] compare the shoulder to the handle of a whip lashing the forearm and hand. There is a rapid internal rotation of the humerus just prior to release of the ball (Fig. 7). This rotation is accelerated by the torque produced by the weight of the ball at the end of the lever arm created by the flexed elbow (Fig. 8). This torque produces the fracture, invariably spiral oblique. The fact that 4 of the 6 fractures occurred throwing a heavier softball lends further support to this hypothesis.

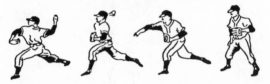

FIG. 7. Illustration of the delivery of the ball by a baseball pitcher. Note the rapid internal rotation of the humerus just prior to the release of the baseball.

SUMMARY

Six cases of ball throwers fracture illustrate the circumstances surrounding this traumatic lesion in healthy young men who participated in athletics to varying degrees. Although always spiral and oblique, with or without comminution, the fracture is not located in any one anatomic area of the humerus, *i.e.* the spiral groove. We see no evidence that the fracture is caused by fatigue or repeated mechanical stress.

The patients had nothing in common other than the mechanism of injury. Considering the frequency with which the action of ball-throwing is repeated, we are unable to explain the relative rarity of this fracture.

REFERENCES

1. Bateman, J. E.: Athletic injuries about the

shoulder in throwing and body-contact sports, Clin. Orthop. 23:75, 1962.

2. Callender, C. L.: Surgical Anatomy, ed. 3. Philadelphia, W. B. Saunders Co., 1942; p. 205.
3. Conwell, H. E., and Reynolds, F. C.: Key and Conwell's Management of Fractures, Dislocations and Sprains, ed. 7. St. Louis, The C. V. Mosby Co., 1961; p. 432.
4. McLaughlin, H. L.: Trauma. Philadelphia, W. B. Saunders Co., 1959; p. 277.

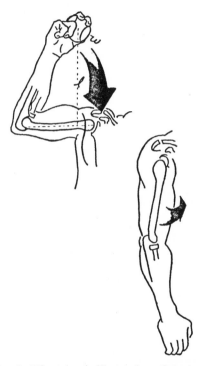

FIG. 8. Diagramatic illustration of the internal rotation torque (w X 1) on the shaft of the humerus during the act of throwing the ball.

5. O'Donoghue, D. H: Treatment oi injuries to Athletes. Philadelphia, W. B. Saunders Co., 1962.
6. Rachun, A., Allman, F. L., Blazina, M. E., Cooper, D. L., Schneider, R. C., and Clarke, K. S.: Standard Nomenclature of Athletic Injuries. American Medical Association, 1966; p. 57.

7. Scudder, C. L.: The Treatment of Fractures, ed. 10. Philadelphia, W. B. Saunders Co., 1926; p. 274.
8. Slocum, D. B.: The mechanics of some common injuries to the shoulder in sports, Amer. J. Surg. 98:394, 1959.
9. Watson-Jones, R.: Fractures and Joint Injuries, ed. 4. Baltimore, Williams & Wilkins, 1952.

Shoulder Injuries in Athletics [*]

MARTIN E. BLAZINA, M.D.

Rather than attempt an academic discussion of orthopedic entities about the shoulder region, this presentation will be limited to injuries unique to athletics, especially those which present difficulties in diagnosis and treatment. Included will be a discussion of some new techniques of radiological investigation, a review of the basic maneuvers of physical examination, and routine x-ray views.

SHOULDER SEPARATIONS (ACROMIOCLAVICULAR JOINT DISLOCATIONS)

On the basis of past experience, two types of acromioclavicular (A-C) joint injuries may be delineated, depending upon the degree of injury to the coracoclavicular ligaments. An incomplete separation implies that these ligaments are still in continuity, whereas a complete

[*] Presented before the Section on Athletic Medicine, American College Health Association, Forty-fourth Annual Meeting, Sand Diego, May 3, 1966.

91

separation indicates significant disruption of these ligaments. A radiographic technique which helps in making this differentiation is the upright view of both A-C joints, with and without ten-pound weights in the hands. In complete separations, the coracoclavicular distance is widened and the clavicle is markedly elevated above the acromion.

In recent years, various examiners have noted an injury to the A-C joint in which the clavicle is displaced posteriorly and not upward. Clinically, the patient experiences severe discomfort near the spine of the scapula. The backward displacement may be difficult to palpate and A-P views may reveal no upward displacement of the clavicle. The A-C joint itself, however, will look wider than usual in the xray film. Treatment of the condition, if detected early, consists of a reapproximation of the joint and holding it in normal position for six weeks. If diagnosis is delayed, degenerative changes occur rapidly in the A-C joint, and removal of the distal end of the clavicle may be required.

In the age group with which we are mainly concerned, complete A-C separations should be treated vigorously by whatever means one thinks effective. In our experience, we have not had great success with slings, casts, or taping and, therefore, prefer open reduction and internal fixation with removal of the fastening device after six weeks. Among the possible complications of internal fixation are loosening of screws, breaking of wires and calcification of ligaments.

SHOULDER DISLOCATIONS AND SUBLUXATION

Everyone is familiar with the classical, frank anterior dislocation of the shoulder, and anyone working with athletes is aware of the strong tendency for these dislocations to recur. In fact, if there have been as many as three episodes of dislocation, corrective surgery is advised, especially if the athlete intends to continue in competition or to remain active in any type of sport.

Radiologically, stereoscopic views, transthoracic or axillary views, and internal and external rotation views will reveal some of the stigmata of recurrent dislocations, such as, humeral head defects, irregularity of the glenoid rim, and loose bodies. Radiopaque arthrography may reveal enlargement of the capsule, avulsion of the glenoid rim, and concomitant tears of the rotator cuff.

Recurrent anterior subluxation of the shoulder, although common in contact sports, is not always well identified by athletic examiners. The condition is quite disabling for football players and it requires the same corrective surgery as recurrent anterior dislocation of the shoulder. In his history, the athlete will usually describe an external rotation injury, such as is often sustained in arm tackling, and a feeling that his shoulder "slipped out," but not completely out. Subsequently, he will have noted recurrent episodes of "slipping out," with spontaneous relocation, followed by aching and soreness in the shoulder and temporary disability.

On examination, he will resist external rotation, and sometimes it is possible to rock the humeral head onto the glenoid rim and feel it slip back. Radiological examinations, as outlined above, may reveal evidence of instability of the shoulder.

Posterior dislocations and subluxations, both primary and recurrent, are extremely rare, but should be kept in mind. An axillary view is extremely useful in detecting a posterior dislocation. If the athlete is able to subluxate his shoulder voluntarily, a cineradiograph will help to avoid confusion about whether the subluxation is anterior or posterior.

PATHOLOGY INVOLVING THE LONG HEAD OF THE BICEPS TENDON

A. *Bicipital Tenosynovitis*

It is our belief that the common condition of "glass arm" in baseball pitchers, resulting in tenderness and pain over the anterior aspect of the shoulder after throwing, represents an irritative tenosynovitis of the long head of the biceps tendon. The rolling of the tendon under the examiner's fingers causes extreme pain. External rotation may also be painful. Our treatment has consisted of heat, local injection of corticosteroids, and judicious resumption of normal pitching activity.

B. *Recurrent Subluxation of the Tendon of the Long Head of the Biceps*

Unlike bicipital tenosynovitis, which usually has an insidious onset, recurrent subluxation of the long head of the biceps tendon is usually associated with some type of injury, incurred either while throwing or while raising the arm overhead against a force (as in water polo or volleyball). The athlete feels a click or slipping anteriorly, accompanied by pain when throwing a ball, especially with the arm in external rotation. The examiner may palpate the subluxating tendon, while maneuvering the shoulder. Unlike cases of recurrent subluxation of the shoulder, the athlete is not quite as apprehensive about being placed in extreme external rotation. Xray views showing the bicipital groove may reveal a shallow groove or an area of soft tissue calcification about the groove. Radiopaque arthrography may reveal that the tendon is displaced from the groove. The treatment is the same as for rupture of the long head of the biceps tendon, as will be described.

C. *Rupture of the Long Head of the Biceps Tendon*

The end result of prolonged, irritative bicipital tenosynovitis or recurrent subluxation of the biceps tendon is rupture of the long head of the biceps tendon. Although this complication is more common in older age groups, it does occur in young athletes, especially in gymnasts who work on the rings. Although the ensuing disability is not overwhelming, the condition should be definitively treated in the young athlete. Our procedure of choice is tenodesis of the tendon into the proximal portion of the humerus. Excision of the intra-articular portion of the tendon should be performed. Otherwise, there will be a bothersome "clicking" of the shoulder and posteriorly-referred pain.

INJURIES TO THE ROTATOR CUFF

Degenerative conditions related to the rotator cuff (calcific supraspinatus tendinitis and subdeltoid bursitis) are not common in the young athlete. It would be interesting, however, to know how many persons in the older age group could associate the onset of this particular shoulder problem with participation in athletics.

Massive ruptures of the cuff are occasionally seen, especially in wrestlers. The resulting inability to abduct the shoulder, the tenderness localized over the subacromial region, and ensuing supraspinatus or infraspinatus atrophy can lead to a clinical diagnosis. Radiopaque arthrography, properly performed, will establish the diagnosis with certainty. The treatment is surgical repair.

The "strained" shoulder seen in football players probably represents an incomplete tear of the rotator cuff. Arthrography does not show extensive extravasation of the dye, as in a significant tear. Treatment is conservative; complete recovery may, however, be prolonged.

NERVE INJURIES

A. *Axillary Nerve Palsy*

In football or other contact sports, the axillary nerve may be injured at its point of entry into the quadrangular space. Deltoid atrophy and "shoulder patch" hypesthesia are clinical manifestations of this problem. Electromyography will substantiate the diagnosis and serial studies will aid in ascertaining the progress and degree of recovery. The treatment is essentially conservative. The prognosis after surgical repair for a complete avulsion of the nerve is poor.

B. *Serratus Anterior Palsy*

"Winging of the scapula" is occasionally seen after a violent stretch injury in wrestling and other contact sports. It is important to examine the posterior aspect of the shoulder girdle in every athlete with a shoulder problem. Pain on movement of the shoulder may be a significant complaint in such cases. Serial electromyograms depict the degree of recovery, and recovery may take a considerable period of time—up to two or three years.

C. *Cervical Root Syndromes—"Pinched Nerve"*

Any problem about the shoulder region presenting with pain and muscle weakness, without a clear-cut history of direct injury to the shoulder, requires an intensive investigation of the cervical spine. Examination of reflexes and xray study to detect narrowing of intervertebral spaces are necessary. Electromyograms may reveal the correct level of the injury. Cervical myelography may reveal a herniated intervertebral disc. Treatment, of course, should be directed toward the neck and should usually be conservative, although an intractable or profound problem may require operation.

RUPTURE OF THE PECTORALIS MAJOR

Rupture of the pectoralis major does sometimes occur in gymnasts and volleyball players. The obvious defect over the anterior chest wall and the pain near the intertubecular groove aid in the diagnosis. If seen early, the treatment is surgical and a good result may be expected If seen late, perhaps, the best treatment is reassurance and regimen of exercise.

RETROSTERNAL DISLOCATION OF THE CLAVICLE: A REPORT
OF FOUR CASES AND A METHOD OF REPAIR

M. A. SIMURDA, M.D., F.R.C.S.[C]

THE sternoclavicular joint is the sole articulation between the shoulder girdle and the trunk. The enlarged sternal end of the clavicle fits in a socket formed by the saddle-shaped facet at the upper angle of the manubrium and the adjacent part of the first costal cartilage. The bony and cartilaginous surfaces of this joint fit poorly, but the interposed fibrocartilaginous articular disc, which divides the joint, makes them congruous. This disc and the anterior and posterior sternoclavicular and costoclavicular ligaments give the joint stability.

Despite this weak anchorage of the shoulder girdle to the trunk, injuries, and particularly dislocations, of this joint are uncommon. Retrosternal dislocation of the clavicle is rare. Rowe and Marble,[1] in an analysis of 1603 shoulder-girdle injuries over a 15-year period, found only 10 sternoclavicular joint injuries. In only one of these was the dislocation posterior. To date, only 51 such cases have been described.[2] In 1963, Tyer, Sturrock and Callow[3] published an extensive review of this injury and its complications. The purpose of this paper is to report four more cases and describe a method of management.

CASE REPORTS

Case 1.—In 1964, N.F., a 15-year-old boy, was tackled while playing rugger. He hit the ground with the lateral aspect of his left shoulder. Immediately, he had severe pain about this shoulder and experienced a "choking feeling" at the base of his neck anteriorly. In the emergency department he was unable to move his left arm and had to support it with his right hand. He held his neck flexed to the left side. His left shoulder was held forward and the inner end of the clavicle was extremely tender. Plain radiographs of the clavicle and sternum (Fig. 1) showed no obvious osseous injury. On examination, the tenderness was localized to the sternoclavicular joint, the landmarks of which were obliterated by swell-

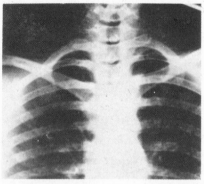
Fig. 1.—Usual anteroposterior view of the sternoclavicular joints shows no definite abnormality.

ing. On palpation, the inner end of the clavicle was no longer in its normal relationship to the manubrium. Tomograms clearly showed that the inner end of the left clavicle was displaced posteriorly and superiorly (Fig. 2).

Under general anesthesia, traction on the arm in various positions of abduction and extension did not reduce the dislocation. The sternoclavicular joint was then opened. The inner end of the clavicle had dislocated in a posterosuperior direction through a tear in the posterior capsule. The cartilaginous cap of the inner end of the clavicle was avulsed but was still attached to the manubrium by the articu-

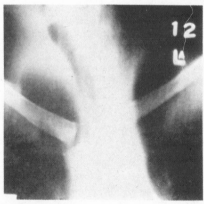
Fig. 2.—Tomogram clearly shows a posterior dislocation.

lar disc. The clavicle was reduced by strong traction on the abducted arm and on the clavicle with bone-holding forceps, but the reduction was not stable. It was stabilized by suturing the tear in the posterior capsule and the articular disc (with the attached cartilaginous cap) to the inner end of the clavicle with heavy silk passed through a drill hole in the upper medial corner of the sternal end of the clavicle. This was reinforced by fixing, with an additional heavy silk suture, the intact sternal head of the sternomastoid tendon to the anterior aspect of the inner end of the clavicle. This reconstruction overcame the posterosuperior instability of the inner end of the clavicle. When the repair was completed, the shoulder could be moved freely without any tendency to redislocation. Using a Velpeau bandage, the arm was immobilized on the chest wall for four weeks. The boy recovered a full range of painless movement and has no disability.

After our experience in this first patient we used the same method of repair in Cases 2 and 3. In this method, the sternoclavicular joint is opened through an incision passing along the proximal two inches of the clavicle and curving gently downwards across the sternoclavicular joint onto the manubrium for a distance of one inch. The dislocation in the younger age group appears to be between the medial end of the clavicle and its cartilaginous cap. In the older patient, the separation is between the medial end of the clavicle and the articular disc. The method of repair is the same in both. The dislocation is reduced by pulling on both the abducted arm and the clavicle itself. The defect in the posterior capsule is closed by a heavy silk suture. The articular disc is reattached to the clavicle with a heavy silk suture through a drill hole in the upper corner of the medial end of the clavicle. The reduction is further stabilized by fixing the intact tendinous sternal portion of the sternomastoid to the anterior aspect of the clavicle with a second heavy silk suture. The arm is immobilized in a Velpeau bandage for four weeks.

Case 2.—In 1964, R.C., a 19-year-old boy, blocked an opposing football player with his right shoulder. Upon impact he felt severe pain in his shoulder and neck, and was unable to move his right arm. He was dyspneic and

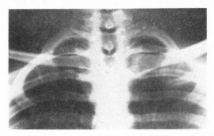

Fig. 3.—Anteroposterior view suggests slight asymmetry.

had a feeling of pressure at the base of his neck. On examination, his right shoulder was held forward and his neck was flexed to the right side. The right jugular vein was distended. He could not move his shoulder because of extreme pain. The sternoclavicular joint was extremely tender and the inner end of the clavicle could not be felt in its normal relation to the manubrium. Plain radiographs (Fig. 3) suggested asymmetry and tomograms readily revealed the posterior dislocation (Fig. 4).

As in Case 1, an attempt at closed relocation was unsuccessful. At operation, the dislocation was seen to be between the medial end of the clavicle and the articular disc. The posterior capsule was torn. The operative repair described above was done and the arm immobilized for four weeks. Within a short time, complete function returned and this young man now has no disability.

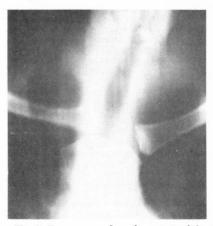

Fig. 4.—Tomogram confirms the posterior dislocation.

99

Case 3.—In 1966, E.C., a 15-year-old boy, received a body check on his right shoulder while playing hockey. He had immediate severe pain at the base of his neck on the right and anteriorly. This was associated with a feeling of pressure in his throat. Because it increased the pain, he could not move his right arm or shoulder. He held the tip of his shoulder forward and his neck flexed to the right side. He was extremely tender over the sternoclavicular joint. The inner end of the clavicle could not be palpated in the normal relationship to the manubrium. Plain films did not clearly demonstrate the lesion but tomograms revealed the posterior displacement.

Closed reduction under anesthesia failed. At operation, the medial end of the clavicle had separated from its cartilaginous cap and dislocated posteriorly leaving the cap and the articular disc attached to the manubrium. At operation, as described above, the dislocation was reduced and stabilized. After four weeks' immobilization, function of the shoulder was restored completely. This boy now has no disability.

Case 4.—In 1967, G.S., a 37-year-old man, was driving a car and was involved in an accident. When seen in the emergency department he complained of severe pain over the inner end of his left clavicle. A hollowness was felt over the sternoclavicular area, and the inner end of the clavicle was not in its normal relationship to the manubrium. Plain films showed nothing, but tomograms revealed posterior displacement. Under general anesthesia, the dislocation was reduced by traction on the abducted arm. The reduction was stable, suggesting that the tear in the posterior clavicle may have been smaller than in the first three cases. The arm was immobilized for four weeks and he has had complete recovery of function without residual disability.

DISCUSSION

All these patients had severe disability and pain. All had symptoms or signs of pressure on the trachea but had no serious complications following the retrosternal dislocation of the clavicle.

The mechanism of injury in all four cases was a strong force transmitted indirectly from the point of the shoulder down the shaft of the clavicle. Forward displacement of the shoulder permitted posterior rotation of the inner end of the clavicle during which the costoclavicular ligaments acted as a fulcrum. When the force is sufficient, the ligaments and capsular structures are disrupted and the inner end of the clavicle dislocates retrosternally. As was suggested by Paterson,[4] the direction of the dislocation may be determined partly by the orientation of the articular planes.

The diagnosis is a clinical one. In all our patients, the direction of the displacement of the inner end of the clavicle was difficult or impossible to determine from the plain films. Tomography, however, helped to determine the degree and the direction of the displacement.

By manipulation, Ferry, Rook and Masterson[5] successfully reduced such dislocations in five patients. We did not have their success; open reduction was necessary in three of our four patients. In the majority of the cases reported in the literature, operative reduction was necessary; these reports stress the difficulties of closed reduction.

In the two 15-year-old patients in this series, the cartilaginous cap covering the inner end of the clavicle remained attached to the articular disc; the disc, in turn, remained attached to the manubrium. In the third patient, a 19-year-old man, only the articular disc remained attached to the manubrium; the inner end of the clavicle with its cartilaginous cap was displaced posteriorly through a tear in the capsule.

We have described a simple method of repair that gives satisfactory results. We had no complications. Others have used intramedullary wires, wire loops and fascial slings in such repairs.[6-9]

SUMMARY

Four patients had retrosternal dislocation of the clavicle. Open reduction was necessary in three. At operation the posterior capsule was repaired with a heavy silk suture passing from the articular disc (with or without the attached cartilaginous cap) to the inner end of the clavicle. Further stability was provided by sewing the sternal portion of the sternomastoid tendon to the anterior surface of the clavicle. This repair was stable and was followed by complete recovery of function.

The author would like to thank Dr. J. W. Hazlett for his permission to use Case 4 in this presentation.

REFERENCES

1. Massachusetts General Hospital, Boston, Fracture Clinic: Fractures and other injuries, by the members of the Fracture Clinic of the Massachusetts General Hospital and of the Faculty of Harvard Medical School, edited by E. F. Cave, The Year Book Publishers Inc., Chicago, 1958, p. 258.
2. LUCAS, G. L.: Retrosternal dislocation of the clavicle, *J.A.M.A.*, **193**: 850, 1965.
3. TYER, H. D. D., STURROCK, W. D. S. AND CALLOW, F. M.: Retrosternal dislocation of the clavicle. *J. Bone Joint Surg. [Brit.]*, **45B**: 132, 1963.
4. PATERSON, D. C.: Retrosternal dislocation of the clavicle, *J. Bone Joint Surg. [Brit.]*, **43B**: 90, 1961.
5. FERRY, A. M., ROOK, F. W. AND MASTERSON, J. H.: Retrosternal dislocation of the clavicle, *J. Bone Joint Surg. [Amer.]*, **39A**: 905, 1957.
6. NIESSEN, H.: Zur Behandlung der retrosternalen Luxation der Clavicula, *Dtsch. Z. Chir.*, **231**: 405, 1931.
7. KENNEDY, J. C.: Retrosternal dislocation of the clavicle, *J. Bone Joint Surg. [Brit.]*, **31B**: 74, 1949.
8. BROWN, R.: Backward and inward dislocation of sternal end of clavicle. Open reduction, *Surg. Clin. N. Amer.*, **7**: 1263, 1927.
9. STEIN, A. H.: Retrosternal dislocation of the clavicle, *J. Bone Joint Surg. [Amer.]*, **39A**: 656, 1957.

Severe Brain Injury and Death Following Minor Hockey Accidents:

The Effectiveness of the "Safety Helmets" of Amateur Hockey Players

JOHN F. FEKETE, M.D., M.C. Path.

IN February 1968, in the snow-bound mining town of Minto, New Brunswick, a 16-year-old high school student was roughly body-checked in a pick-up hockey game by an opposing player much bigger than he. He fell and hit his left temple on the ice. Even though he wore a protective helmet, he never regained consciousness, but developed fixed dilated pupils and died within two hours in the ambulance on his way to hospital in Fredericton.

From the Regional Laboratories and Victoria Public Hospital, Fredericton, New Brunswick.
Presented at the 1968 Annual Meeting of the Canadian Association of Pathologists, Banff, Alberta, June 12-15, 1968.

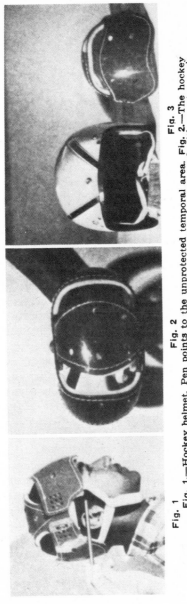

Fig. 1   Fig. 2   Fig. 3

Fig. 1.—Hockey helmet. Pen points to the unprotected temporal area. Fig. 2.—The hockey helmet is easily compressed by one hand. Fig. 3.—A hockey helmet compared with a motor-cycle helmet. The motor-cycle helmet is obviously stronger and has a suspension gear. It is heavier and more cumbersome.

Two-and-one-half months later, another 16-year-old high school student, while playing in the Eastern Minor Tournament in Oromocto, New Brunswick, was hit on his right temple by the hockey stick of an opposing player. Although he wore a protective helmet, he suffered a broken skull, soon lost consciousness and died with fixed dilated pupils within six hours.

This was the third death of the 1967-68 hockey season, if we include that of Bill Masterton of the National Hockey League, Minnesota North Stars, who died on January 13, 1968, in a game against the Oakland Seals.[1]

In the medical literature there are apparently no statistics available regarding head injury and death attributable to hockey.[2] In the New Brunswick daily press, however, there is a reference to a previous death due to ice hockey. A New Brunswick man of 21 died 28 years ago after striking the back of his head on the ice while playing in minor league hockey.[1]

Both New Brunswick players who died this season were protected by helmets. This fact naturally focused attention on the adequacy of the protective equipment of hockey players, especially of the helmets.[3] The protective head gear of an amateur hockey player is a rather flimsy affair which, in many cases, instead of protecting the head, appears to invite carelessness, and violence on the part of the opposing players (Fig. 1). The usually ill-fitting helmet protects only the upper part of the skull. It gives somewhat better protection if the fit is right. Being made of thin plastic material, however, it does not have enough rigidity to give adequate protection against any but the slightest blow. The type of helmet used by the players who died could be compressed easily by one hand (Fig. 2). It is lined by a thin layer of plastic foam approximately 3/8" in thickness and it does not have suspension gears. In comparison, the motorcycle or football helmet has a rigid shell and a suspension gear (Fig. 3). The football helmet covers most of the head and gives adequate protection from the type of injury that proved fatal in the two cases described above. If it is not worn properly, however, even the motorcycle helmet leaves the vital and weak temple area unprotected.

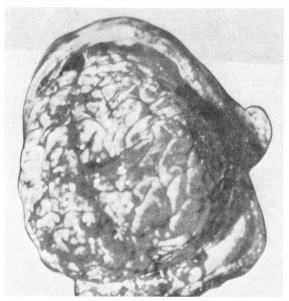

Fig. 4.—Case 1. Brain *in situ* showing diffuse subarachnoid hematoma.

In our first case (R.R., aged 16) most of the positive postmortem findings were in the head. In the left temporal muscle a recent hemorrhage was present. The bones of the skull, however, were intact, as was the dura mater. The brain weighed 1600 g. and was edematous. Beneath the dura, a thin layer of fresh blood covered both cerebral hemispheres. Some

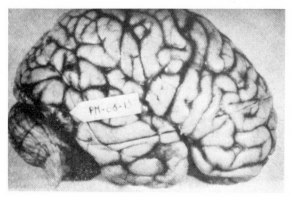

Fig. 5.—Case 1. The brain showing diffuse subarachnoid hemorrhage and contusion of the occipital cortex.

of this hemorrhage was subarachnoid, but the larger portion was subdural (Fig. 4). Some of the free blood seeped down along the spinal cord, as far as the mid-thoracic segments.

The gyri of the brain were flattened, but there was no evidence of temporal lobe herniation. The cerebellar tonsils were herniated into the foramen magnum. On the lateral margin of the right occipital lobe there was a soft, hemorrhagic surface contusion 1 x 2 cm. in size (Figs. 5 and 6). Two smaller contused hemorrhagic areas were also present; one on the lateral edge of the right temporal lobe measured 1 x ½ cm. and the other on the upper aspect of the cerebellum close to the midline measured only ½ x ½ cm.

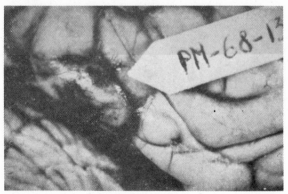

Fig. 6.—Case 1. Close-up of the contusion on the right occipital lobe of the brain.

Section of the brain disclosed several slit-like hemorrhages in the pons and in the cerebral peduncles (Fig. 7).

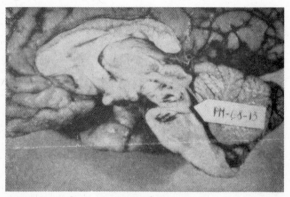

Fig. 7.—Case 1. Sagittal section of the brain. Streak-like hemorrhages in the brain stem.

In the fatty connective tissue behind the left eye was a hemorrhage which showed through the thin bone of the orbit and presented as a bluish discoloration underneath the left upper eyelid.

The blood vessels of the brain were all thin-walled, obviously patent and well formed. The circle of Willis was intact and no aneurysms or arteriovenous fistulas could be found.

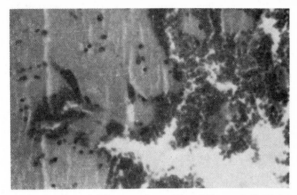

Fig. 8.—Case 1. Microscopic section of the occipital lobe of the brain showing the contusion and hemorrhage. Note the absence of cellular reaction. (H.E. stain, × 250 magnification.)

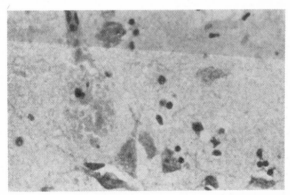

Fig. 9.—Case 1. Microscopic section of the brain stem showing a small hemorrhage. The nerve cells show loss of tigroid granules. (Nissl stain, × 250 magnification.)

The rest of the autopsy showed only petechial hemorrhages of the larynx and trachea with very marked pulmonary edema and hemorrhage.

Microscopic examination of the brain showed necrotic tissue and small streak-like hemorrhages in the area of the contusion on the occipital lobe (Fig. 8).

The large nerve cells in the immediate area were distorted and showed neuronolysis; at the periphery of the lesion they were unremarkable. There was no evidence of cellular reaction in this area. Sections taken from the smaller contusion on the right temporal lobe showed similar changes, without cellular reaction. In the subarachnoid space there was a large number of red blood cells with occasional mononuclear cells or polymorphonuclears.

The hemorrhagic areas in the pons and in the cerebral peduncles showed demyelinization of the white matter around the hemorrhagic area, loss of nuclear staining and tigroid of the nerve cells, with complete cytolysis in a few areas. Many polymorphonuclears and a few glial cells were seen in and around the hemorrhages (Figs. 9 and 10). The contused area of the cerebellum was rather superficial, involving mainly the grey matter, and already a number of polymorphonuclears and an occasional mononuclear cell could be seen. The Purkinje cells had completely disappeared (Fig. 11); In the sec-

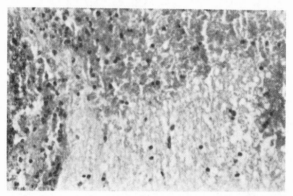

Fig. 10.—Case 1. Microscopic section of brain stem showing larger hemorrhage with infiltration of leukocytes and edema. (H.E. stain, × 100 magnification.)

tions taken from the bruise and contusion of the left temporal muscle the muscle fibres could be seen separated by red blood cells, but there was no evidence of cellular reaction or phagocytosis.

In our second case also (E.G., aged 16), apart from moderate lung edema, the pathological changes were confined to the head. The scalp showed abrasions of the skin over the right temple and in front of the right ear, measuring ½″ x ¼″ and ⅛″ x ⅛″ respectively. The whole right temporal area was swollen by a hematoma of the right temporal muscle. When the temporal muscle was reflected,

108

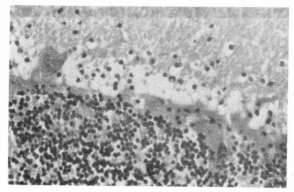

Fig. 11.—Case 1. Microscopic section of the cerebellum showing the disappearance of the Purkinje cells. (H.E. stain, X 250 magnification.)

a fracture in the right temporal bone was detected. The fracture was depressed about ⅜″ and formed a three-sided flap almost rectangular in shape. The superior and posterior lines of the fracture crossed the branches of the right middle meningeal artery, resulting in an epidural hematoma of dark red, soft, jelly-like consistence. The volume of the hematoma was 3 oz. The brain showed edema with flattening of the convolutions and narrowing of the sulci. A moderate cerebellar cone was present.

On the lateral aspect of the right temporal lobe a recent cortical contusion 1½″ x 1½″ in size was apparent, together with hemorrhage. There was flattening of the right temporal lobe due to the overlying epidural clot and causing distinct asymmetry of the cerebral hemispheres. In addition there was fresh subdural blood clot spread over the right

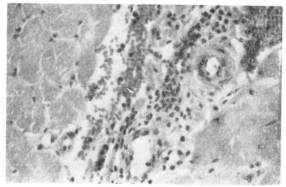

Fig. 12.—Case 2. Microscopic section of the right temporal muscle showing the hematoma with many leukocytes. (H.E. stain, X 100 magnification.)

temporoparietal area, extending forward to the frontal lobe and measuring approximately ½ oz. in volume.

The cerebral vessels were healthy, and serial sections of the brain showed no other focal injuries. The cerebellum and brain stem were normal, apart from edema.

Histological examination showed necrosis, infiltration with polymorphonuclears and hemorrhage at the site of the injury in the temporal muscle (Fig. 12). There was evidence of recent cortical contusion in the right temporal lobe of the brain without glial, mononuclear or polymorphonuclear cellular reaction. The epidural clot consisted of a red thrombus with occasional aggregates of leukocytes and scanty hematoidin granules.

DISCUSSION

In Case 1, death was due to multiple closed brain injuries. Histologically these injuries could be divided into two distinct groups, depending on their age. To the group of more recent injuries belong the contusion over the right occipital lobe (contrecoup) and the one over the right temporal lobe (intermediary coup). Microscopic observations, using the criteria set forth by Lindenberg and Freytag[4] (Table I), placed the contusion of the cerebellar cortex and the hemorrhages in the brain stem in a second group of injuries of longer duration. The advanced degenerative and reactive changes indicated that this second group of injuries was at least a few days old and could not have been sustained at the time of the fatal hockey game. Our observations and conclusions were supported by the testimony of a witness who saw the deceased fall and hit the back of his head on the ice four days before the fatal accident. At that time he briefly lost consciousness and probably sustained tiny, slowly expanding hemorrhages in the brain stem and in the cerebellum, causing weakness, unsteadiness and headaches. When, during the fatal hockey game, he was roughly body-checked by a much bigger player, he could not protect himself and just "flopped" down, hitting his left temple hard against the ice. This would explain the severity of his brain damage and also the temporal muscle hemorrhage in an area protected by the helmet (Fig. 13).

In Case 2 the cause of death was a fractured temporal bone with underlying epidural and subdural hematomata and cerebral contusion. The deceased was hit by a hockey stick on the right temporal area. This area was not protected by the helmet (Fig. 1). The contusion of the brain was a primary coup type of injury. As expected in brain injuries caused by blows, there was no contrecoup injury (Fig. 14).

TABLE I.—Time-Table of Microscopic Changes in Cerebral Contusion

(Modified and tabulated after Lindenberg and Freytag[4])

I.—Phase of Necrosis

Less than 1 hour:
  Extravasation of red blood cells. Elongation and shrinkage of nerve cells in the centre, vacuolization on the periphery.
3-5 hours:
  Secondary extension of hemorrhage. Edema. Polymorphonuclears appear in subarachnoid space.
24 hours:
  Shrunken nerve cells become pale and show chromatolysis. Glial cells are pyknotic. Early demyelinization of white matter is seen.
36 hours:
  Complete disappearance of nerve cells in the centre; incrustation of pericellular structures in the border zone. Polymorphonuclears may appear in the deeper necrotic areas.
48 hours:
  First gitter cells appear in white matter (microglia). Mesodermal cells in leptomeninx are swollen.

II.—Phase of Resolution

2-4 days:
  Gitter cells and histiocytes appear in large numbers (compound granular cells).
4-7 days:
  Marked proliferation of vascular, glial and white blood cell elements forming a granular layer around the necrosis.
2-4 weeks:
  Marked proliferation of granulation tissue. Early lytic changes.
1-2 months:
  Lytic changes progress. Early cyst formation.
2-4 months:
  Well-formed cysts.

A witness testified during the inquest that the deceased was hit by the tip of a hockey stick

111

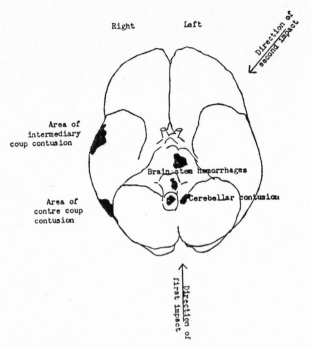

Right   Left

Direction of second impact

Area of
intermediary
coup contusion

Brain stem hemorrhages

Cerebellar contusion

Area of
contre coup
contusion

Direction of
first impact

Fig. 13.—Case 1. View of lower aspect of brain showing contused or hemorrhagic areas with reconstruction of impact forces.

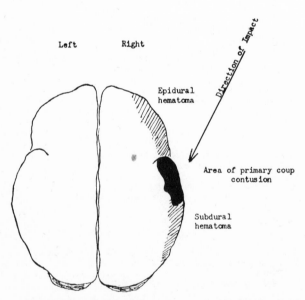

Left   Right

Direction of Impact

Epidural
hematoma

Area of primary coup
contusion

Subdural
hematoma

Fig. 14.—Case 2. View of upper aspect of brain showing contused and hemorrhagic areas with reconstruction of impact force.

112

after a scuffle behind the net in a "deliberate attempt to hit high in a blind anger", while skating away from the site of the incident.

A hockey stick swung with full force travels with a high velocity, it weighs approximately 1½ to 2 lbs. and it can hit with an estimated kinetic energy of 72 foot-pounds.[5] In our case, the full energy and impact force of the blow was concentrated into the tip of the hockey stick, less than 1 sq. cm. in area. A force of this magnitude would probably be sufficient to impress the weak temporal squama even if it was covered by the thin plastic helmet.

Lindenberg and Freytag[6] classify the mechanisms of cerebral contusion in three large groups:

1. Cases with impact to the movable, not accelerated head (blows).
2. Cases with impact to the accelerated head (falls).
3. Cases with impact to the supported head (crushing injuries).

With blows, one usually finds only a primary coup type of injury. Because of the slow deceleration of the skull, no contrecoup injuries are seen; Case 2 belongs in this category. With falls, primary coup injury is uncommon, but one can expect to see marked contrecoup injuries caused by the sudden deceleration of the skull; Case 1 belongs to this group. Obviously in hockey injuries one cannot expect to find cases of the third type, the crushing injuries.

The ideal protective hockey helmet, therefore, should be able to protect the players against blows and falls. The shell and the suspension apparatus of the helmets should be able to cushion enough of the impact of falls and blows to reduce the transmitted accelerating or decelerating velocity of the head below the 30 ft. per second danger threshold found by White and associates, and below the 425 lbs. per sq. in. pressure found by Gurdjian.[7] Apparently 30 ft. per second is the upper limit of impact velocity which the human brain can suffer without experiencing cerebral concussion. Likewise, 425 lbs. per sq. in. is the approximate upper limit of pressure which the human skull can withstand without fracture.[7]

The helmet should also be light and compact in size to avoid adding further weight to the already top-heavy human head and to avoid shifting the centre of gravity upward and forward, thereby increasing the moment of inertia about the cervical pivots, which would in turn increase the sheer stresses and create whiplash effects at the moment of impact.[7] It is known that whiplash injuries of the head can produce subdural hematomata and brain contusions without an actual impact to the head.[8]

Summary Two teenage hockey players died in New Brunswick as a result of brain injury suffered while playing minor-league hockey. Both players wore hockey helmets. The first was body checked and fell. He suffered several contusions of the cerebral cortex and hemorrhages in the brain stem without fracture of the skull. His condition was aggravated by previous minor head trauma. The second player was hit by a hockey stick and suffered a depressed fracture of the right temporal bone with cerebral contusion and hemorrhage. It is emphasized that: (1) the so-called protective helmet of amateur hockey players gives only limited protection, even in minor accidents; and (2) a minor brain concussion with loss of consciousness may set the stage for subsequent lethal brain damage, even in the absence of skull fracture or epidural hematoma. Further experimental studies are being planned in collaboration with the Department of Mechanical Engineering of the University of New Brunswick, Fredericton, to measure certain features of the protective hockey helmets in view of their lack of effectiveness in preventing brain damage.

REFERENCES

1. *The Telegraph Journal (Saint John)*, February 14, 1968, p. 3.
2. ROWLAND, M. L. (Prior Information Research Service) : Personal communication.
3. *The Daily Gleaner (Fredericton)*, May 6, 1968, p. 9.
4. LINDENBERG, R. AND FREYTAG, E.: *A.M.A. Arch. Path.*, 63: 23, 1957.
5. CAMPBELL, J. S., FOURNIER, P. AND HILL, D. P.: *Canad. Med. Ass. J.*, 81: 922, 1959.
6. LINDENBERG, R. AND FREYTAG, E.: *A.M.A. Arch. Path.*, 69: 440, 1960.
7. OMMAYA, A. K.: *Ann. Roy. Coll. Surg. Eng.*, 39: 317, 1966.
8. OMMAYA, A. K., FAAS, F. AND YARNELL, P.: *J. A. M. A.*, 204: 285, 1968.

HEAD AND NECK INJURIES IN ATHLETES

NEAL I. ARONSON, M.D.

Dr. Richard Schneider, chief of neurosurgery at Ann Arbor, has been interested in football injuries for a long time. He has published some interesting statistics. If anyone wants the references I will be glad to furnish them.

On the other hand there are some who have made the point that the face mask for instance, one of the recent acqusitions in football, may actually, while it is protective to the face, the nose, and the jaw, be detrimental to the neck. It has been shown experimentally that the further the face mask protrudes in front of the face the more of a lever arm it constitutes, in the event a player is struck with an upward blow in the face mask, it causes about double the amount of force that would ordinarily be generated by a blow on the jaw. In other words, if a man has his head in the extended position and he's struck on the face mask from the front, he gets about a hundred pounds or more of force transmitted to the upper cervical spine, and then if he has a relatively small head and a large helmet on, the back part of the helmet can catch him in the suboccipital region

Presented at Seminar on the Medical Aspects of Sports, August 14, 1967.

and create enough strain so that under severe circumstances a fracture dislocation of the cervical spine might occur. This is an area I believe that needs further scientific investigation.

Another traumatic factor perhaps is the helmet itself. With the advent of very hard plastic helmets there has been some suspicion that there is transmission of force to the skull, directly from the helmet, whereas in the older days the softer helmets caused the force to be dissipated. It is interesting to note that you do not have to produce a direct blow to the head in order to produce internal injury to blood vessels and brain and it would seem again that if some way could be developed to cause a spreading of the force rather than a direct head-on propagation from the helmet to the skull, this would be helpful.

I realize that there is a webbing inside the helmet but it does not seem to dissipate the force as well as ideally we would like it to do, and some intelligent engineer will have to work on this problem which is beyond the scope of the doctor's training to really investigate.

In one type of research, transducers are being placed into helmets during actual games in order to find out how much force is transmitted to the head through the modern hard plastic helmet.

Another thing that you have read about I am sure in the newspapers recently, and is of some importance in reference to head and neck injuries is the habit of "spearing" or "butting" an opponent. It seems that Dr. Schneider did an investigation of this and found that in the western colleges they teach this as a standard operating procedure in football. He finds, when he analyzes his data of serious and fatal injuries to the head and neck of which there are quite a few every year, that there seems to be a direct correlation between this type of tackling and serious injuries to the ncek and head. A recent plea has been made which was published in the *JAMA* that this type of tackling be abandoned in football and that it actually be penalized. I think I would have to agree with that conclusion.

I will begin by reviewing a little anatomy of the head and neck and then go on to discuss some of the symptoms of different types of head and neck injuries. Before doing so I think I would like to make the general plea that when a patient has a head or neck injury whether he complains merely of headache or dizziness or whether he complains of pain or stiffness of the neck, pain down the upper arm, extremities, numbness, or what have you, that the trainer think in terms of appropriate consultation before allowing the palyer to resume competition. These conditions are a little more subtle and more difficult to diagnose and are potentially more dangerous than simple sprains, strains, bumps and hematomas, bruises, and simple extremity fractures.

If a person has an injury to the neck, the simplest form is a sprain and this can be produced usually by sudden flexion or extension of the head particularly if the head is partially rotated when the force of the blow is sustained.

Football is a dangerous sport. There is no question about that, and as we get larger and larger antagonists in the game especially in the professional ranks, the amount of force that is brought to bear on the player becomes extreme. Therefore it is important to stress that people who are in this type of activity be first of all highly conditioned athletes and take regular calisthenics to keep their muscles in the best possible state of tone. That in itself is as important a preventative of injury as I know.

And secondly a man has to learn how to run. If a man for instance, is the ball carrier it has been shown that the safest running position is with his head in neutral position, perhaps flexed slightly at the waist but not flexed or extended at the region of the neck or with his head turned markedly to one side or the other. Naturally it is impossible even when rushing not to look for the hole in the line to get through but a man should train himself so that when he is actually getting into the opposing tacklers that his head return to normal alignment and that he maintain his muscles in a state of tension. \There are some arguments concerning the danger of keeping the muscles tense when being tackled. It may actually provoke the fracture of long bones or extremity bones but it difinitely protects the spine.\ I think that highly developed back and abdominal muscles and neck muscles will prevent injury to this area of the anatomy. Keeping the head from being turned markedly to one side or the other, extended or flexed, will also prevent this type of injury as much as it is possible to do.

If there is an injury, the simplest form of injury I mentioned is a sprain and this is merely a tearing of a muscle or the ligamentous attachment of a muscle and it produces stiffness, tenderness, and some swelling locally, unassociated with any neurological symptoms. This is treated by the trainer usually with heat, usually moist heat, muscle relaxants, and rest. Rest is extremely important. Immobilization in the collar is usually not necessary for simple strains.

Occasionally when there is an injury to the neck it may be accompanied by neurological symptoms or signs and this becomes a more serious injury. For instance, the patient may complain of sudden numbness in one or both arms or his lower extremities, or he may demonstrate some weakness in the distribution of his muscles. If this is transient one can assume that the patient has merely had what we call contusion of the spinal cord. But in order for a contusion to occur there has to have been enough tearing of important ligaments arund the vertebrae to allow one vertebra to slip slightly on another or subluxate.

Now such a patient should be examined by a specialist either in orthopedics or neurosurgery and have X-rays made of the cervical spine. This is extremely important. I don't think any patient who has a neurological symptom should ever merely be treated conservatively and sent back to his duties without having films made and a consultation. I would think that if there is any persistence of symptoms such as in the case of Paul Hornung that the man should not be sent back into the lineup with one of these balloon collars appended to his uniform but should be kept out of competition for the rest of the season. I feel that this is a potentially very serious type of injury.

We rarely, see more serious injuries to the cervical spine where there is an actual fracture and one vertebra is displaced upon another. Such a patient usually has clearcut neurological problems in addition to an extremely painful stiff neck which he is unable to move. If a patient is injured in this region of his anatomy and is lying on the football field complaining of severe pain in his neck, numbness, or inability to move his extremities, he should be moved only with the utmost caution by skilled personnel. At least five or six people should put him on a stretcher and his head should be maintained in slight traction at the time that it is done and then he should not be moved again until he is brought directly to a specialist with X-ray facilities.

Fortunately, it is very hard to produce an injury of the intervertebral disc in a normal young person. Disc injuries do occur in football but are much more common as you get into the older age groups. The men who have been in professional ball for several years and are getting up into their mid thirties are the ones that are most subject to disc injuries because a normal disc in a healthy young person is actually stronger than the bone which surrounds it. It has been shown experimentally that if you take a spine and place it in a vise, (the normal spine of a young person who has died for instance, in an automobile accident or some other cause), and put pressure on the longitudinal axis of that spine you will fracture a vertebra before you will rupture a disc.

There are some people who are subject to early disc degeneration and these people usually give the clue of having had either neck ache or backache intermittently rather early in life. People who have postural problems or people who complain of having had backache in the past, of sciatica in the case of lumbar disc, that is, pain going down the leg or pain into the region of the

119

shoulder blade or down the arm should be seen by a specialist and probably X-rayed before they are considered to be candidates for a football squad.

Disc injuries as I mentioned are rare but we have seen an occasional disc protrusion or rupture due to a sporting injury and the treatment will depend upon the severity. The milder cases are treated by traction and immobilization in a collar followed by a period of physiotherapy. More severe cases are treated by surgical intervention. It is possible for a professional athlete or for a college player to go back after a disc excision. I would not advise it after a neck or cervical disc excision but lumbar disc injuries have resulted in sufficiently good recovery following surgical removal so that these individuals may return to active sports. One of my colleagues here in town, operated on a quarterback from Notre Dame about five or six years ago and he went back the following year and had a very productive season.

The reason for this is that it is safer to operate in the lumbar region because the spinal cord has terminated several inches above where the lumbar disc injury occurs, so that even if there were a recurrence due to a second injury it would not be of serious neurological consequence whereas on the other hand with a cervical disc you have the spinal cord to contend with and a recurrent injury to the neck could result in permanent paralysis, as the physicians at the Mayo Clinic advised Paul Hornung before he retired this year.

Sudden extension injuries or flexion injuries of the neck especially as I mentioned with the head slightly rotated produced the type of sheering force that could produce a fracture dislocation and a potential injury to the spinal cord or vertabral artery. The latter structure runs in a tunnel of bone in the cervical spine.

While on this subject I will mention injuries to the carotid artery. These are the large arteries in the front of the neck, that do not run in bone but do supply the major portion of the blood to the cerebral hemispheres or upper portion of the brain. We know of a few instances of young

120

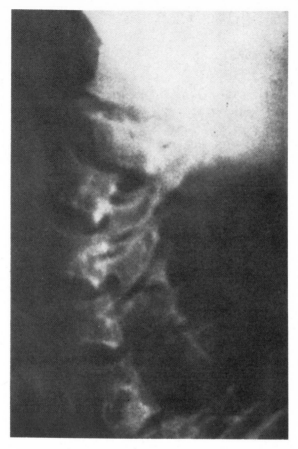

Figure 1
Note the severe fracture dislocation in the lower cervical region, and how this vertebra has slid forward on the other.

people developing a traumatic thrombosis of the carotid artery by a direct karate type chop blow to the neck, and the neck of course, is always to be protected. Again, fouling of an opponent should always be avoided and a man should learn to run so that the front of his neck is in a protected position. The large shoulder guards that are worn today plus the proper position of the neck will tend to prevent an injury to the carotid artery.

Here is an example in Figure I of the injury

121

that can be caused by hyperextension of the neck with sudden blow to a face mask. This is a fracture dislocation of (45) the upper cervical region, potentially a fatal injury.

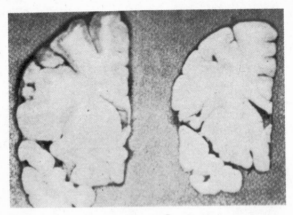

Figure 2
A section of the brain at autopsy showing cerebral edema. The left side indicates the portion most severely swollen.

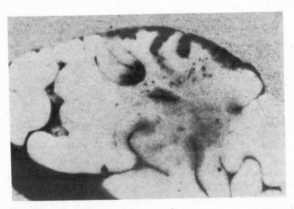

Figure 3
A hemorrhage brain. An autopsy specimen showing the hemorrhages under the cerebral cortex.

Here is a severe fracture-dislocation in the lower cervical region. Note that this vertebra has slipped forward on the other. This patient of course was quadriplegic. This was not a football injury.

The man was paralyzed at the moment of impact (I believe this was a diving accident, a very common cause of this type of injury) in all four extremities and was rushed to the hospital and immediately put in skeletal traction which is where we put the so-called "ice tongs" in the skull in order to reduce this fracture and put it back into normal position. Later when the spine was examined surgically the spinal cord was found to be torn which if course meant that the patient would not recover any useful function. It is very rare to see this type of injury as a result of football, but it does occur.

According to a recent survey, head and neck injuries constitute only a very small percentage of football injuries but they account for about 80% of the deaths, so you realize that we are talking about a very important and critical portion of the anatomy.

Here in Figure 2 is brain which is swollen. This is a section of the brain at autopsy due to what we call cerebral edema, the result of a severe concussion. The left side indicates the portion that is most severely swollen. This is due to a collection of fluid which comes out of the capillaries and fills up the intercellular spaces of the brain.

Here in Figure 3 is a brain that has actual hemorrhage in it. This is referred to as a cerebral contusion. Note the little hemorrhages under the cerebral cortex in this autopsy specimen, and also the little petechial hemorrhages around the blood vessels.

Again it is interesting to note, that the sandlot player who does not have proper equipment would be the man you would think most subject to injuries of this magnitude, but this does not prove to be correct. Looking at the statistics you will find that the most severe injuries of the head and neck occur in the professional athlete, and I think this is directly related to the force at which these men hit and their body weight. They are now getting up into the behemoth size weighing 275 to 300 pounds and can hit with the force of a frieght train. The college athlete is second on the list. The high school athlete actually has one of the lowest rates of severe injury of this kind and I believe it is because they play a cleaner game even though they may not have as much finesse as a professional and because of the fact that we are dealing for the most part with men of more average body weight and size.

Let us turn to head injury for just a moment. I haven't discussed that in any detail. There are several gradations of head injury.

The first and most common thing that you will observe on the football field is the man who is just slightly dazed as the result of a play. If this lasts only for a few seconds and he immediately comes back to his senses I see no reason why this man should not be allowed to continue in the game provided he has no other complaints. But if the man becomes confused, and we have seen this on many occasions, he should be taken out of the game and be sent for a specialist's examination within a reasonable period of time.

In order to make the diagnosis of cerebral concussion which is (aside from scalp lacerations and abrasions and contusions) the first type of brain or head injury that we have to take into consideration, it is necessary to dicit a history of unconsciousness and a period of retrograde amnesia. This means that the individual was definitely "out" even if it was only for a few seconds, that he has difficulty remembering what transpired just prior to the time he was hit, or his memory may be entirely foggy for the period just before and just after the time that the play was run. A man who has had a concussion should be taken out of the game and regardless of how well he says he feels he should be examined by a specialists.

A man who complains, following a head injury, of persistent headache, or dizziness, of ringing in

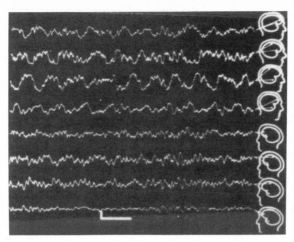

Figure 4

the ears, or shows confusion, falls into this category and requires further elucidation. In addition to taking a history and doing a careful neurological examination I think an electroencephalogram is worthwhile. This can show us subtle degrees of brain injury.

Here is an example in Figure 4 of an electroencephologram showing slow-wave activity over the left side of the brain in a person who sustained unilateral hemorrage and edema following a blow to the head. In less severe injuries more subtle changes can be seen.

Now I think a man who has been seriously enough injured to produce changes in the electroencephalogram probably should be kept out of action for the rest of the season because there is a statistical chance that such a man might get late complications such as convulsive disorder or epilepsy as a result of a bad enough contusion of the brain. It is true that this rarely occurs but I think that one has to respect the brain as a very sensitive organ which is easily damaged and if the individual has shown unconsciousness, retrograde amnesia, perhaps some minor neurological changes, persistent dizziness, ringing in the ears, confusion, or anything like that, plus some irregularity in electroencephalogram, that man is entitled to be out of action for the rest of that season in my opinion.

Now the next type of brain injury I would like to mention is more severe and fortunately quite rare: is extradural hematoma. This is usually due to usually a fracture through the squamous portion of the temporal bone.

It is a well-known fact that blows to the temple are potentially fatal and this is the explanation (although there are other reasons). When the bone is fractured in this area—and usually this type of injury can only occur when the helmet has come off or when for some reason the man hasn't worn one and then receives a direct blow to the side of the head—the middle meningeal artery which is the artery that supplies the covering of the brain, the dura, can be torn because this artery runs through the bone before it gets to the brain and it runs through the bone precisely in this region, the temporal squamosa.

This of course, bleeds vigorously when it is torn because it carries arterial blood. Arterial blood is circulated under a much higher pressure than venous blood and therefore a collection of arterial blood develops over the membrane which surrounds the brain and creates pressure on the brain.

The characteristic picture of this injury is that the patient complains of excruciating headache after an initial period of unconsciousness and then gradually begins to lose consciousness again. Accompanying this there is is weakness usually of the opposite side of the body. And there may be dilatation of the pupil on the side of the injury due to pressure on the oculomotor nerve, which runs past the area involved to go on the eye.

This combination of findings constitutes a neurosurgical emergency. Six such cases were reported over a five-year period which was reviewed by Dr. Schneider in 1964 and five of them died. Theoretically, most if not all of these could be saved by early surgical intervention and that is why, if a man shows progressive changes of severe excruciating headache following a head

126

injury he should immediately be taken to a specialist.

The next type of injury I would like to mention is the so-called subdural hematoma which is a hemorrhage beneath the membrane surrounding the brain but still outside the brain.

There was a time when we thought that injuries of this kind mainly occurred in infants or in aged people and especially in alcoholics. The reason for the latter is in early youth and late in life the brain tends to be smaller than the skull and there is more than a potential space in which bleeding can occur. However even young adults can develop subdural hematoma and in this survey conducted by Dr. Schneider which I previously alluded to, it was the most potent and most frequent serious brain injury that was seen in football players. They had some 65 cases of subdural hematoma with an appallingly high mortality rate. One of the reasons that the mortality rate was high in this group was because the acute subdural hematoma often had some arterial bleeding associated with it. The chronic subdural hematoma, the symptoms of which come on gradually over a period of a couple of weeks, is usually due to venous bleeding. Veins of course carry blood under low pressure and they tend to bleed only until they are tamponaded by their own outpouring of blood and then the bleeding stops, whereas arterial bleeding will go on more rapidly and more extensively. On the other hand, many of the subdural hematomas discovered were probably in the subacute or chronic category and these patients too could have been saved with appropriate and early diagnosis. Many of them were. But invariably some are lost.

The commonest reason for this is that in many communities specialized services are not available and this is a field in which only the neurosurgeon can participate because there is no other field that consists in dealing with diseases of the brain per se in a surgical sense. The general surgeon however who goes through a good program has had some experience in rotating through the neurosurgical training and should have the ability at least to diagnose and in some instances even to drill small openings which we call trephinations to relieve the acute pressure of subdural bleeding. Unfortunately, not all general surgeons have had such training.

If a man has a severe head injury he should be transported as soon as the local doctor feels his condition will permit to where specialized care is available. There are many diagnostic tests and tools that are available in large medical cents to facilitate the diagnosis of these conditions without doing exploratory surgery. In most instances it will be found that the man does not have such a severe injury but it is much better to err on the side of safety than to overlook an injury which might later prove to be fatal. In subacute or chronic subdural hemaloma the situation is less urgent. The patient may seem a little woozy and groggy and be confused just as though he had a simple concussion and then feel fine for several days, but a week or so later he may start suffering from headache and periods of somnolence, ability to concentrate and may then begin to show some weakness on one or both sides of his body or some double vision When these symptoms have their advent it is the time to immediately seek consultation.

Occasionally, a man will die suddenly after a blow on the head. Some of these deaths are due to massive hemorrhage from a ruptured aneurysm. This is a congenital abnormality which weekend a blood vessel in the brain. according to an autopsy survey this is one of the rarest causes, as is brain tumor, of sudden death due to head injury. The majority of them are due to garden variety type of head injuries most of which are theoretically if not actually treatable by proper diagnostic studies and early surgical intervention.

Skull fracture itself, which I mentioned before, does not necessarily have to be a very serious type of injury but it is indicative of the force of the blow which the individual sustained and it indicates the necessity of a careful observation of that patient for complications such as intracranial bleeding. Many types of skull fracture are simple: they are not depressed; they are not comminuted; they are not compounded. In other words, there is no indriving of dirt because there is no overlying laceration in the majority of instances and they are not pushed into a position where they create pressure on the brain. These may just be treated by simply watching the patient until they heal. I would think that a man who has had a skull fracture, regardless of how simple it might be in its appearance, should be out of action for the rest of that year.

Athletic Head and Spinal Injuries

JACQUES E. BOTTON, M.D.

IN THIS ERA of strong emphasis on physical fitness among the young and also among the not so young, injuries associated with all kinds of athletic activities have become increasingly more frequent. Physical fitness has almost become a slogan with social, educational, and even political overtones at times. Increasing emphasis brings increasing participation as well as interest in all its phases. Injuries resulting from these activities must therefore be well understood, not only by the physician, but also by all members of groups participating in such activities. No doubt, prevention would be the preferable and the most efficient way to deal with them. However, the subject of this presentation is most specifically directed toward the handling of an injury affecting the head as well as the

Presented by invitation at the Conference on Medical Aspects of Sports, Charlottesville, July 21, 1968.

spine in the first few minutes and hours following the accident. Specialists in various fields of medicine have learned to work as a team when an individual is brought to the emergency room of a well equipped hospital. In most cases, when the extent of the injury is not well known from the very onset, a general surgeon usually heads the team, progressively turning over to the appropriate specialist the handling of a specifically more important injury.

There seems to be a particular mystery that somehow shrouds the handling of head and spinal injuries, not only among laymen, but also for many physicians. The knowledge of a few simple principles very often clears the picture adequately to allow good handling of the problem.

I am not aware of an athletic activity completely devoid of possible danger. The direct body contact or the impact from falling and striking the ground is one of the most common factors in injuries in football. Baseball not infrequently will expose a player, or even at times a bystander, to the blow of a pitched ball or the bat itself. Boxing needs very little emphasis as to the kind of blows exchanged towards victory, and the press has frequently brought news of a particularly fatal ending to such events. Javelin, as well as the discus, may produce penetrating wounds of the skull, and more rarely, of the spine. Serious injuries have not infrequently resulted from a golf ball hitting an unexpected human target. Similar injuries may very well occur in squash, either with the ball itself or the racket. Ice skating, basketball, and other activities will result in injuries from falling on the ground. In 1961, Schneider, from the University of Michigan, presented statistics relating to the death of fourteen players from injuries to the brain or spinal cord occurring in 1959 as recorded by the "Serious Injuries and Fatalities Committee of the American Football Coaches Association". Actually, there were 208 fatalities from either head or cervical cord injury reported to this group in the period from 1947 through 1959.

Head Injuries

Let us first consider some phases of head injuries that may result from the above mentioned athletic activities.

Anatomically, the head is a closed, spherical, bony cage that somehow manages to balance itself over the cervical portion of the spinal column, and containing as well as protecting a most sensitive, vital, sophisticated organ. The most elaborate computer equipment available to industry today is unable to come close in performance to that of a few cerebral cells. This bony cage is covered with a well vascularized scalp separated from it only with a very thin, but very richly innervated and therefore sensitive membrane, the periosteum. Scalp lacerations, therefore, are usually associated with fairly extensive bleeding, as well as pain arising from the injured periosteum. ·

The skull itself can be subjected to mainly two kinds of fractures: a linear fracture, which is simply a hair-line separation without loss in the curvature of the skull itself. Not infrequently, multiple linear fractures may be present and rather irreverently the term "egg shell fracture" is used to illustrate the findings on x-ray. It is interesting to note that head injuries due to a same degree of blow are less serious when associated to a skull fracture than otherwise. Most of the force seems to be absorbed by the fracturing of the skull and less is transmitted to its contents with less chance, therefore, of direct injury to the brain itself. There should be little concern, therefore, for the skull fracture per se. The complications that may go along with it are what we really worry about. A linear fracture most of the time brings about nothing more than a headache of a few hours to a few days' duration, but careful observation in a hospital with specialized medical personnel available is indispensable. Occasionally an artery will have been interrupted by the fracture, with formation, fairly rapidly, of a blood clot between the bone and the underlying membrane that covers the brain, the dura mater. This results in the so-called epidural or extradural hematoma. The individual may be awake for one to several hours and then quite rapidly lapse into unconsciousness, weakness on the opposite side, a dilated pupil, respiratory difficulties, etc., necessitating a very prompt surgical precedure for evacuation of the clot as well as the occlusion of the bleeding artery. This is the kind of head injury most frequently responsible for death following a direct blow to the head in boxing, baseball, etc. Even when the surgeon is able to evacuate the blood clot, stop the bleeding, and eventually prevent death, full recovery may not result. There may be residual paralysis, speech impairment, as well as intellectual deterioration.

The second type of skull fracture is known as a depressed skull fracture; it may or may not be associated to a laceration of the scalp over it, in which case it will be grouped under the name of compounded and depressed skull fracture. Unless such a fracture damages a large vessel, artery or a venous sinus, there is no definite urgency in surgical repair. It is preferable to give attention to whatever other injuries the individual may have and bring him to an optimum general condition before going ahead with the operation.

Most of the time, however, head injuries will not necessarily be associated with a skull fracture. The impact in these cases is directly transmitted to the brain itself and more serious complications may occur. Transient loss of consciousness, even of a few seconds, followed by complete recovery except for slight headache or dizziness, is the result of a brain concussion which is a very short-lived arrest in the cortical activity with no permanent damage to any part of the brain. When such damage does occur with some residual remaining, such as weakness, loss of memory, loss of speech, etc., then the term brain contusion is used. A more extensive amount of brain damage can be due to a laceration of the brain itself with or without hemorrhage within its substance. Injuries of this type are associated with increasing degrees of swelling of the brain just like any other organ that has been injured. However, the space within the skull being definitely limited to the volume of the brain, any increase in its bulk will endanger its function, particularly when one considers that it will ·also slow down its blood supply and oxygenation with further production of edema in a vicious cycle. Therefore, not all head injuries followed by loss of function or consciousness are necessarily due to bleeding and the formation of an intracerebral or intracranial clot or hematoma.

How should we, therefore, watch an individual who has just been subjected to a head injury? What are the most important signs or symptoms to look for in order to give appropriate care?

It is rather simple. The most important thing to watch is the state of consciousness. We personally do not like to use words such as coma, semi-coma, stupor, etc., which do not always mean the same thing to everybody. It is best perhaps to describe reactions of the individual to his surroundings. The cerebral activity, when not allowed to go on normally, will result in decreasing degrees of awareness. The patient may be fully awake, well oriented in time and in space, alert, immediately following a blow to his head. Only in the subsequent minutes or hours would he slowly become drowsier, less active and responsive to questions. Or he may have been immediately rendered unconscious following the blow and remain so subsequently. This is most important and worthwhile noting, whether by the other team members, coach, the ambulance driver, or the nurse at the emergency room. Immediate and lasting loss of consciousness means immediate and serious brain damage due to cerebral swelling as well as hemorrhage within it. Whereas a progressive decrease of mental capacities towards complete loss of consciousness would be more in keeping with a developing subdural or epidural hematoma for which much more can and should be done as soon as possible. It will therefore be very helpful to the physician to know the individual's state of consciousness immediately following the injury.

The single most important advice, therefore, would be to observe the patient's alertness and response to questions and report immediately to the physician when this response becomes less easily obtained. Other symptoms and signs are known to be suggestive of increasing intracranial pressure, but I would like to re-emphasize that they are by far less important and useful than the state of consciousness. With the intracranial pressure increasing, the pulse rate slows down while the blood pressure increases, as the heart has to work harder to push the circulating blood through the cerebral vessels. Nausea and vomiting may occur, respirations may become irregular, and at late stages stop altogether. The pupil on one side, then the other, may dilate and be non-reactive to light. Hemorrhages may be seen within the eyegrounds. Epileptic seizures may occur and one side become weaker than the other, and so on. But most of these signs are rather late or difficult to observe by the layman.

A brief loss of consciousness may sometimes be associated with loss of spontaneous breathing. This usually is due to a concussion, with momentary decrease in cerebral activity, but no evidence of organic injury to the brain. The player should immediately be given artificial respiration and, unless a serious degree of brain contusion has occurred, he will be able to breathe again and awaken. He should then be allowed to slowly raise himself and should he again begin to faint, placed recumbent and withdrawn from the game. However, if he does feel well and is able to sit without discomfort, he may sit on the bench, but should be observed for the following minutes and hours. Of course, any scalp laceration that may have occurred will be taken care of. Unless an extensive amount of blood has been lost from a large scalp laceration, shock or hypotension is almost never due to a head injury, and if this occurs, injury elsewhere should be suspected, such as a ruptured intra-abdominal organ, etc. Only after the cause for shock has been discovered and corrected should the head injury problem be considered and managed.

When the individual who has just been hit on his head has either remained, or become unconscious shortly after the injury, an adequate airway must be immediately obtained and maintained. It is useless to administer oxygen while, because of massive facial injury or swelling around the neck, etc., the patient is unable to receive it into his lungs and use it properly. The airway will be obtained either by a mouthpiece, or in more advanced stages a tracheotomy urgently performed and in these cases, definitely life saving. Suction will allow clearing of the upper respiratory airway; loose teeth or dentures should be removed, particularly when there is a tendency to vomiting. The patient should be turned on his side and slightly facing down in order to prevent further embarrassment of the airway by his vomitus. Quite often an airway will be improved by extending slightly the neck while pulling on the jaw.

The basic advice given to medical personnel in emergency rooms in the handling of head injuries is listed: 1. Establish a clear airway, 2. Treat shock, 3. Conduct a complete physical examination.

Once the airway has been obtained in an adequate fashion, the shock treated, and the patient examined, ancillary studies are available and frequently necessary to make a complete evaluation of the patient's head injury. Simple x-rays of the skull will demonstrate the extent and location of fractures and, particularly in cases of linear fractures and in individuals who are otherwise alert, warn towards the possibility of a developing extradural hematoma in the ensuing few hours. Hospital observation in these cases is definitely indicated. Special studies may then be carried out if the patient's condition allows. A recent device is the ultrasonic encephalogram. It helps detect any shift of the midline structures within the head to one side or the other as a result of a developing intracranial hematoma. Angiography, which visualizes the intracranial vessels by injection of a radiopaque material in the carotid artery in the neck, may suggest the location and the extent of a clot. Quite often, however, the physician is unable to carry out all these studies and his hand is forced into performing exploratory operations, namely burr holes, towards the discovery of a clot and its removal.

As mentioned above, head injuries, often may not be associated with any skull fracture and yet be serious enough to impair the patient's awareness, produce paralysis, or even epileptic convulsions. This is due either to simple swelling of the entire brain or to associated hemorrhages within its substance. This can occur immediately, in the following few hours, or sometimes three or four days after the initial injury. The above mentioned studies will help rule out a developing clot and these patients can then be treated by drugs capable of decreasing the amount of swelling (steroids, urea, mannitol). Occasionally, an individual who did well for several days or weeks following an injury may show signs of progressive neurological malfunction with resulting headaches, mental dullness, etc., and he will be found to be suffering of a subdural hematoma or hydrocephalus. This again will warrant careful observation by the physician. It is very unusual that this will occur beyond a few months following the injury.

An individual may have been subjected to a head injury mild enough to cause nothing more than a certain amount of headache and dizziness. This may last for several days, may or may not be associated to nausea and vomiting. It is usually important to reassure him that no serious complications have occurred and that recovery should be expected within a few days to a week. He will usually respond fairly well to rest, mild analgesics, etc. We do not believe that he should be allowed to participate in the usual athletic activities until he has fully recovered from the above mentioned effects of the head injury. Some individuals will tend to minimize while others will exaggerate their difficulties and this, of course, will require good insight into that particular individual by his family, his coach, as well as the physician himself.

Spinal Injuries

Let us now consider injuries that may involve the spinal column. For clinical purposes, the spine is divided into three main segments: cervical, dorsal and lumbar. The cervical spine is by far the most mobile and, therefore, most readily exposed to injury. Besides its role in supporting the body and allowing man to be an erect animal, the spine also contains and protects the spinal cord. It is very strongly supported by a multitude of sturdy ligaments and muscles which are very intimately inter-related. Injuries to any part of the spine, therefore, will affect muscles, ligaments, the spinal column, or the spinal cord itself in various combinations.

The most simple and benign injury will result in contusion of the muscles close to the spine at various levels with or without involvement of the intervertebral ligaments. The neck as well as the low back are more frequently involved, with resulting stiffness and pain of various degrees. Rest and immobilization of the involved levels, as well as mild pain medication, usually suffices to bring about a fairly rapid recovery. At times heat and application of traction may also be necessary. We believe that pain is a protective symptom that should be respected rather than ignored if more serious complications are to be avoided. This, of course, applies to all phases of medical management. Whether contusion involves the neck or the low back, an underlying injury to the spine itself should be ruled out with adequate x-ray studies and further follow-up. A more severe degree of injury is muscular and/or ligamental strain of the neck or lumbar area and would necessitate a more prolonged period of recovery and treatment. Most of the time an adequate degree of traction, particularly when the neck is involved, becomes necessary, following which the individual may have to wear a protective collar for several days or a few weeks. Traction seems to be less effective when the other parts of the spine are involved and would only result in keeping the patient in bed which is, of course, the main point of management.

A rather common occurrence in association to contusion or strain of the cervical or lumbar spine is a herniation of an intervertebral disc with subsequent pressure on a nearby nerve root producing severe pain and numbness as well as weakness of an arm or a leg on the same side. This may happen within a few days or sometimes several months to a few years after the original injury, following a definite weakening of the spine itself. After a reasonable period of conservative management involving bed rest, physical therapy, and other means, not infrequently surgery becomes necessary in order to prevent further disability as well as loss of function in terms of weakness and numbness of an extremity.

Injury to the spine can, of course, result in a fracture with or without dislocation. When the spinal cord is not involved paralysis does not occur and the patients eventually recover after a lengthy medical management that may at times require a surgical reduction of the fracture and fusion of the involved level in order to prevent further difficulties. The problem becomes most critical at the cervical spinal level where a subsequent injury may then involve the spinal cord itself with serious complications, such as paraplegia or quadriplegia. It is important to remember that a fracture-dislocation following an injury may, after careless manipulation, result in injury to the spinal cord secondarily, with paralysis developing quite rapidly at that time.

When an individual has injured his spine, he should not sit up, but rest on his back and keep immobile. If he is awake, it will be most important to see whether he can move his arms and legs and breathe without difficulty. The location of the pain should also be noted. If the neck seems to be involved, the head can easily be immobilized by putting sandbags on either side or by gentle traction in the direction of his body applied under his chin and the back of his head. Whenever feasible, a physician should immediately examine the player on the spot, even if this requires delaying the game for several minutes. Only then should he carefully be moved to an adequate stretcher, producing as little motion of the patient's body as possible. The recent introduction of a two part metal stretcher that fits under the patient from either side and locks, has been a welcome addition to the equipment of life saving crews. If the individual is also unconscious, or even simply drowsy, the care should be multiplied as he would be unable to indicate the exact location of his suffering and maintain his airway.

The head, neck, and shoulder form a triangle which very frequently is involved in various combinations of its components. Whenever two of these elements are involved, the third should be strongly suspected of having been injured as well. For example, if there is evidence of injury to the head and shoulder, one should be very certain that the neck has not also been involved. This will, of course, avoid unnecessary manipulations with further complications. Neck injuries will occur in a variety of fashions. Acute extension or hyperflexion, forceful rotation of the head to one side, can all result in serious injuries. A particular concern has arisen from the head gear worn in football. There is no doubt that this piece of equipment gives definite protection against head injuries. However, by its very rigidity, it becomes a hazard when the neck is thrown in hyperextension with the back of the helmet against the spine, resulting in injury to the spinal cord as well. A new helmet has the plastic back of the neck cut away and replaced with an apron so that it is impossible for the edge of the plastic to impinge against the neck proper. A strip of plastic foam beginning at the forehead and extending up over the crown of the helmet and about six inches wide, serves as protection for the opposing player. It also has plastic pads inside. Some players have complained of this being somewhat hotter, but it certainly seems to be more protective. The single face bar for protection has in some cases been replaced by double ones which do not extend as far forward and reduce the leverage to some extent. They are harder to grasp because of the spread between the bars. The blocker is also less likely to get his elbow, shoulder, or knee under the bars since the lower one is considerably further towards the chest. Another alternative design has a sturdy extension from the back of the helmet towards the neck following its contour, protecting it from damage by hyperextension.

A not infrequent form of injury involves the sudden stretching of the brachial plexus by forceful pulling on one arm or a fall, putting all the weight on one shoulder. This results in avulsion of the brachial plexus with immediate paralysis or at least marked weakness of the involved arm. The spine itself is usually not involved in any way. These injuries may take several months to recover from and often may not allow full return of function. Adequate padding across the shoulders may decrease this possibility only to some extent.

In closing, we would like to emphasize that while injuries to the head or the spine remain, fortunately, most of the time benign and without serious complications, it is impossible to guess whether a particular incident will remain so or develop into a more major catastrophy. It will therefore be best to "play it safe" and to ascertain as much as possible the exact nature of the injury rather than allowing a player to return to the game towards an early victory and perhaps a delayed defeat. One should also avoid the opposite extreme of overprotecting a child who has suffered, let us say, a moderately severe head injury, from which he has been declared recovered by his physician but who may well become a mental cripple by not being allowed to return to normal activities with his friends and school mates.

THE
FOSBURY FLOP

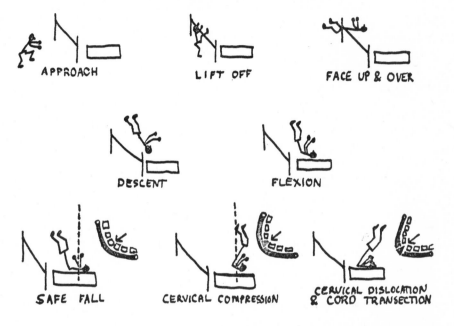

AT THE 1968 SUMMER OLYMPICS in Mexico, the world was amazed at the bizarre style of Bill Fosbury, winning the Gold Medal for the United States in the high jump, going over the bar at seven feet, four and a quarter inches. His self developed style consists of—

1. A strong push-up at the base of the jump.
2. Ascending and rolling his body to the left so that the entire ventral or anterior surface of his body is skyward, or away from the bar.
3. A descent, head first, downward.
4. Flexion of his neck on his chest at a critical time, and the cervical vertebrae absorb the initial force of the fall.
5. At this point his pelvis and lower extremities are swinging in a

wide arc downward, and at the point of the contact of the neck and the landing pad, the pelvis had not passed a perpendicular line from the cervical vertebrae upward. The neck does not absorb the force of the fall.

6. Completion of the jump by the continued wide arc of the pelvis downward, flexing his hips and landing on his back, and finishing the jump on his feet.

The success of the jump depends on the timing of the jumper. The pelvis must not be past the perpendicular line at the point of impact, and the arc must be wide enough to bring the neck out of flexion as the pelvis travels. The pad on which he lands is an expensive air-filled rubber bladder, peculiar to the Olympics and well-endowed colleges. In his hands, the style is safe, successful, and he is certainly a credit to the United States. However, he was seen on television, jumping in his own style, by millions of potential high jumpers and coaches throughout the world, and they were envious that a young boy could develop his own style and win over the most experienced jumpers in the world. You can imagine how many athletes are waiting until springtime when they can experiment with the Fosbury method in their own jumping pits at school. You can also imagine the number of cervical injuries we will see this spring.

THE JUMP AND CERVICAL DISLOCATION

In the hands of the inexperienced high jumper, the Fosbury style is downright dangerous and even death producing. The follies of the style are two-fold. The first folly is the manner of the landing. Most high jumpers go over the bar face down and land on all four extremities, and thus, absorb all shock to the spinal cord and vertebrae. In the Fosbury technique, the actual landing is on the anteriorly flexed cervical vertebrae with the neck in acute flexion. If the pelvis does pass the perpendicular at the exact time of touchdown of the neck, then the body weight will fall on the cervical and high thoracic vertebrae, causing further acute flexion of the vertebrae. The force at this point produces compression of the anterior vertebral body, and as the weight is continued, the vertebral body is dislocated, putting pressure on the spinal cord. If the force continues, the dislocation will produce a transection of the spinal cord with a resultant quadriplegia.

The second folly of the Fosbury style is the pad on which the jumper lands. Without personal knowledge of the pad Fosbury used in training, or the pad used in the Olympics, let us examine within our experience the usual pad used in the better high schools and colleges, and those used by the less affluent schools. In discussing the problem with our local coaches, it was stated that the Olympic pad was a large air-filled bladder, and if this were so, then this appliance is excellent for absorbing the forces of a perfectly executed Fosbury jump. However, even this pad could produce a serious injury if the jump were not perfect. This air-filled bladder is expensive and beyond the funding of most athletic departments.

146

The most common and entirely satisfactory pad for the training of high jumpers is the soft foam rubber mattress about two feet thick. For the conventional classic jump this is quite adequate, but would be deemed far too hard for the training of the Fosbury Flop, and thus the most commonly used pad would become a source of serious neck injuries in the inexperienced jumpers.

Some high schools cannot even afford to buy the two-foot thick foam rubber pad and must resort to the old style method of using discarded bed mattresses. These old mattresses are adequate for landing in the conventional style of high jump, but consider Bill Fosbury landing on one of these hard surfaces. Saw dust is still considered adequate in some schools and there is a lot to be said for it in producing any type of injury. Team physicians are expected to examine these new procedures and techniques with a critical eye and advise the coaches and school authorities as to the dangers of their use. It does not take much of a critical eye to see the dangers of the Fosbury Flop, even if it produces a single Gold Medal winner. In spite of this warning, there will be certain coaches who will encourage the boys to try it and a certain number of transected cervical spinal cord quadriplegics will be produced.

In my experience at a spinal cord center, we are seeing athletes, especially high school athletes, as an increasing source of spinal cord damaged patients. Football has been the primary cause of paraplegia and quadriplegia, followed by diving, gymnastics, and water skiing. Lately, we have added an increasing number of trampoline accidents. Athletics cease to be a sport when you see a number of high school and college boys sitting around in wheelchairs in a paraplegic center.

Therefore, I will call on all physicians, especially team physicians, to bring all the pressure possible on the local high schools and colleges to outlaw the Fosbury Flop. The High School Athletic League Associations should bring this matter to their next meeting before the spring training starts and vote for its elimination as a competitive technique in the classical high jump.

The Fosbury Style of jumping over the high bar is dangerous. This bizarre style of jumping can produce serious neck injuries, including cervical fractures, and permanent damage to the high thoracic and cervical spinal cord. Quadriplegia or death could result from accidents in trying this style of jumping. Every effort should be made by the coaches themselves to control the style of the high jump. High School Athletic League Associations should outlaw the style of the jump at their winter meeting. The Sports Medicine Committee of The Medical Society of Virginia and the American Medical Association should endorse the physical folly of the style and recommend its immediate abolition before spring training begins in 1969.

147

Stress fractures in athletes*

M. B. DEVAS, F.R.C.S.

A STRESS fracture may be defined as that fracture which occurs in the normal bone of a normal individual undergoing normal activity and with no injury. To understand stress fractures, or as they are sometimes called, fatigue fractures, it must be understood that the normal bone of a healthy individual is very much alive and that it is in no way comparable to a concrete post but it is much more like a piece of living wood.

However, in certain respects bone differs from other material to which it might be compared in that it has the ability to restrengthen itself after it has become weakened by use. During use bone absorbs energy; were the bone to be made of metal or concrete it would break in due course of use. But bone, being alive with a free flowing blood supply, normally does not break but continuously regains its lost strength.

Athletes, usually in the full vigour of youth, are essentially fit and do not have abnormalities or disturbances of metabolism but they can, by over-exercising especially when not in training, lay themselves open to an increased incidence of stress fractures. Thus a marathon runner in full training will be less likely to develop a stress fracture at, say, the twentieth mile than another who is out of training. Thus training counts even in avoiding stress fracture, because bone will become stronger by being used, in exactly the opposite way that it becomes weak with immobilization in plaster.

Athletes are not the only people to sustain stress fractures and, using the tibia as an example, out of every 100 stress fractures approximately 36 occur in athletes at about 18 years of age; 23 occur in children of whom some are athletic but not all; and the rest occur in older people, with the exception of a small number in ballet dancers.

Types of stress fracture

In the main, there are two types; one in which the bone is compressed (figure 1) and one in which the bone is bent and thus breaks (figure 2). It is important to emphasize that all stress fractures are caused by muscular activity, or pull, on the bone and they are not caused by heavy footfalls in running or when jumping jars the bone.

Diagnosis of stress fractures

The classical symptoms caused by a stress fracture are that, first, the athlete complains of pain towards the end of his sport, or shortly afterwards, which is described as "a bit of an ache", or "a little nagging pain", but to begin with it is not severe and it does not cause him to seek attention. However, with the continued practice of the sport the pain begins to become not only more severe but also to occur earlier during the sport; it lasts longer and sometimes disturbs sleep. However, next morning the athlete feels better and may be encouraged to start running again only to find that after a short while the pain comes on severely and, although the activity is stopped, the pain remains. Advice is sought and perhaps a week's rest is advised. At the end of that time the pain has gone completely with ordinary activity but as soon as the athlete returns to sport the pain comes on again with renewed emphasis. This pattern of coming on, resting,

*Reproduced by kind permission of the Academic Board of the Institute of Sports Medicine.

148

getting rid of the pain, returning to sport and further pain may be repeated to the detriment of the athlete throughout the season.

The history of the pain is all important because physical signs are not always easily found. In the fibula it is possible, on occasion, to see a little swelling if the stress fracture is in its lowest third (figure 3). However, this particular bone does allow palpation at that area and a swelling may be felt on the bone; it is hard, being of callus or pre-callus, and is fusiform and tender. Springing the fibula from above may cause pain at the

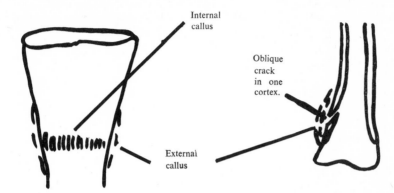

Figure 1.
Diagram of a compression stress fracture.

Figure 2.
Diagram of the oblique stress fracture common to athletes caused by bending of the bone.

fracture site. In the tibia, with 'shin soreness' in runners, there is again local tenderness and a little local swelling may be felt but, in the early stages, swelling of the bone is rare. In any other part affected tenderness will be present but usually it is difficult to elicit accurately because most bones are well covered with muscles. The stress fracture of the metatarsal bone which often occurs in athletes can, of course, be felt in much the same way as the fibula.

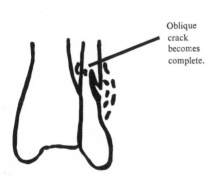
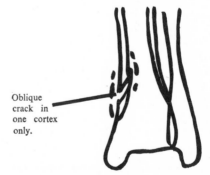

Figure 3.
Diagram of a stress fracture of the lower third of the fibula. Note that there is soft tissue swelling just visible above the lateral malleolus.

Figure 4.
Oblique stress fracture of the tibia which is the cause of shin soreness. Note that the fracture in the lower part of the tibia runs upwards and inwards through one cortex only.

Radiographs are notoriously slow in revealing a stress fracture and up to three months can elapse in certain fractures before confirmation is seen radiologically. Meanwhile, any form of blood test or other pathological investigation will come back with a normal result.

Treatment

This is basically simple but not always easy to carry out. Absolute rest of the part to the extent of not developing the pain must be ensured. Thus the weekend amateur athlete may be allowed to continue his work as a bank clerk provided he takes no exercise. If, however, even this work causes pain, then he must rest at home. Elastic adhesive strapping gives support to the leg and shows the athlete that treatment is being given. But, above all, it is rest which must be prolonged to suit the time for each fracture to unite that cures the lesion. A stress fracture of the tibia may take four to six weeks and occasionally longer before it is united so firmly that training can start with impunity. When there is clinical evidence, through lack of tenderness at the fracture site, that the fracture has united, the athlete is allowed to return to gentle training under careful supervision; provided this does not cause any recurrence of symptoms, training is increased.

It is however, very important to allow the bone time to become strong for the particular muscular activity before it is subjected to complete stress, such as a race or a match.

The common types of stress fracture in athletes

The fibula

The lowermost third of the fibula is the most common site for a stress fracture in athletes and is often known as the runner's fracture. The history is typical of a stress fracture as has been given above and, at this particular site, the clinician is fortunate to be able to feel the bone underneath the skin and the fusiform swelling at the fracture site

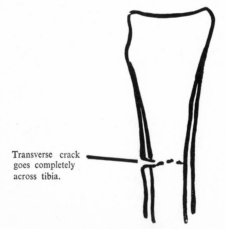

Transverse crack goes completely across tibia.

Figure 5. A transverse stress fracture shown diagrammatically in the centre of the tibia such as occurs in a ballet dancer. This fracture readily becomes complete with continued activity.

can be felt; very rarely it can also be seen. Springing the fibula by pressing upon its shaft above the site of the pain may cause pain at the fracture site. Radiographs will show initially a small oblique crack in the outer cortex of the fibula, running upwards and inwards, about five centimetres above the tip of the lateral malleolus. After a further period of time radiographs will show that the fracture has progressed and gone right across the fibula shaft and that callus is present all round. This is not always the case and, if an athlete stops running as soon as he gets the pain in the lower part of the fibula, the fracture may not progress across the whole of the shaft but may stay confined to the lateral cortex only. The treatment is standard; rest from pain-producing activity and elastic adhesive strapping. Usually the athlete is able to start training, under observation and with care, four to six weeks after treatment has started.

Metatarsal bones

A march fracture occurs in athletes as it does in others and is fairly easily recognized by pain localized to the shaft of one or other metatarsal bones. In this respect, the base of the fifth metatarsal bone can also sustain stress fractures. The first metatarsal bone appears to be exempt in athletes. The radiographs will show the fracture usually to be in the metatarsal neck although occasionally the base of the bone has the fracture. The pattern is similar to that in the fibula in that the fracture rapidly becomes complete across both cortices of the metatarsal shaft. Again, however, if the onset of pain coincides with the cessation of activity the whole of the bone may not break. Rest with supportive bandaging is sufficient to allow healing in four to six weeks but a special note of warning is needed for those stress fractures that occur at the base of the fifth metatarsal bone because here the pull of the tendons may distract the fracture to give a small gap and union can take a long time. Pain may, at times, be severe and when this is the case, a short period in a below-knee walking plaster is useful.

The tibia

The tibia causes more trouble to the athlete than any other bone because of the often insidious nature of presentation of stress fracture. Many other conditions have been evoked to account for shin soreness but with the exception of the anterior tibial syndrome, all forms of true shin soreness are caused by stress fractures.

Classically, shin soreness shows itself as pain in the shin coming on with or after exercise as in other stress fractures. Almost invariably it is only the anteromedial cortex of the tibia that is involved. A short period of rest suffices to ease the pain and the athlete is tempted to return to his sport; in other words, the bone is never given sufficient time to heal and a whole season may pass with interruptions for short periods of rest followed by more training and, in turn, followed by more pain.

Clinical examination will often reveal a tender spot in the tibia and, although the lower third is common, the upper third also sustains the same fracture. Radiographs may show early callus formation only appearing as a small subperiosteal swelling of new bone and sometimes the crack can be seen (figure 4). Rarely the outline of the callus is jagged as though the periosteum has ruptured and the haematoma from the fracture has become ossified outside the periosteum. Radiographs may not show the fracture or the callus for a month after the onset of symptoms and occasionally for longer and on occasion three months is needed for some fractures to show.

Treatment must be rigorous. Rest must be assured for at least a month to six weeks before training is allowed and then very judicious care must be taken to ensure that the athlete tries out the leg before doing anything too active. Thus the best method of testing that a stress fracture of the tibia has united is to let the athlete do simple skipping under controlled conditions for a certain period and, if no pain occurs, to increase that period each day over a week. Should pain occur under the circumstances outlined, the activity is immediately stopped and a further two-weeks rest ordered.

Ballet dancers' fracture

Ballet dancers and occasionally athletes, sustain a stress fracture exactly in the middle of the tibia in its anterior cortex. This is a dangerous stress fracture in that it may allow the tibia to break completely, particularly if activity is continued. This stress fracture will heal quickly under the same regime as for others in the tibia.

The humerus

The upper shaft of the humerus has been known to sustain stress fractures in cricketers, particularly with heavy fielding practice or bowling. Usually, because it is not a weight bearing bone, the aching is accepted by the athlete as muscular until a sudden throw allows the fracture to break the shaft completely and the arm falls useless to the side. Treatment again is simple by restricting the activity of the member concerned. Displacement with the complete fracture does not occur and union is speedy, occurring in a month.

Other stress lesions

Practically any part of any bone in the leg can sustain a stress fracture; the femoral neck, patella, the tibial plateau, the calcaneus and the sesamoid bones are all vulnerable, but fractures are rare in occurrence.

Stress lesions also occur at certain ossio-tendenous junctions such as, in children, the tibial tubercle or the lower pole of the patella; even the anterior and inferior superior iliac spines can be avulsed in whole or in part, as can the lesser trochanter. Avulsions from stress must be distinguished from the avulsions from muscular violence which occur suddenly with one particular movement. The avulsions from stress are chronic and cause pain with activity in just the same way that pain occurs with a stress fracture. However, because they are mostly in children and because they are somewhat outside true stress fractures, further details are not necessary here.

Discussion

The history of a stress fracture occurring in an athlete is usually fairly easily recognized. Sometimes, if the activity is stopped forthwith, the signs and symptoms may settle with no radiographic confirmation. This does not mean that there has not been a stress fracture but that it has been so slight that it has not been seen radiographically. Provided treatment, which is rest from the activity causing pain, is continued and is uninterrupted the fracture will unite and the athlete will return to sport with no increased likelihood of getting another stress fracture than he had initially. It must also be remembered that simultaneous stress fractures of two bones is acceptable because the stress on any one bone should be equalled by the stress in the same bone on the opposite side. However, often one bone is, perhaps, a little ahead of the other on the opposite side in developing the stress fracture and the pain produced in the most advanced side restricts activity so that the lesion is not diagnosed—or even considered—on the opposite side.

Finally, no stress fracture should ever be diagnosed in an unfit athlete without very careful exclusion of all other pathological causes. The peak incidence of stress fractures is from about 16 to 26 years when muscular activity is at its height and physical prowess at its best. But, at the same ages other conditions, although rare, can be found, such as a bone tumour, which can mislead the clinician. Should any bone lesion not behave absolutely typically, it is always wise to advise a biopsy; this will not keep a patient away from sport any longer than the stress fracture from which he is suffering if, indeed, this is still the diagnosis, because the complete rest necessitated heals the fracture quickly.

Evaluation of the Results of Treatment of Soft Tissue Injury

Dr A Zinovieff

The assessment of the results of treatment of soft tissue injury can be made in two ways, through clinical examination and through functional assessment.

In the case of muscle or ligament injury, clinical examination alone can indicate if the treatment has been entirely successful and that the patient is ready for athletic activity. The cardinal signs of recovery following ligament injury are: (1) No tenderness. (2) No pain on stretching the damaged ligament. (3) No laxity, if necessary confirmed by special X-rays with appropriate strains. If these three tests are negative, treatment has been completely successful.

In the case of muscle injury the cardinal signs of recovery are: (1) No tenderness. (2) No muscle shortening and no pain on stretching. (3) No pain on contraction against resistance. (4) No weakness. If these four tests are negative, treatment has been completely successful and the patient is ready to resume athletic activities. The restoration of full length of the injured muscle is important and is sometimes forgotten. Until this occurs some pain will be felt on vigorous use of the muscle, which handicaps the athlete.

Whilst a rough idea of muscle power can be made by using manual resistance and comparing it with the normal side, it is better to demonstrate this more accurately and exactly by using a spring balance. This method is more quickly done and

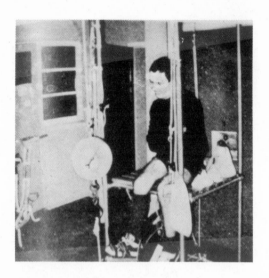

Fig 1 *Measuring the single spring lift*

with less fatigue to the patient than trying to estimate the one repetition maximum (1 RM) recommended by DeLorme (1945). Fig 1 illustrates how a spring balance can be introduced into a pulley and weight circuit to test the power of the quadriceps. Long muscles are most powerful in their middle ranges of movement and the test in the case of the quadriceps starts at about right angle flexion of the knee. The resulting measurement is recorded as a single spring lift (SSL) (Zinovieff 1951). For comparison the SSL is also measured on the normal side.

For some time a relatively expensive stamped commercial type of spring balance, costing over £10, was used (Fig 2) but more recently it has been found that a cheaper, non-commercial model, which costs just under £5, is sufficiently accurate and is smaller, lighter, and thus easier to use.

If these tests suggest that treatment has not been entirely successful and that recovery is incomplete, or in the case of more severe joint injury such as dislocation, functional assessment is required. While this can be fully done only in a gymnasium under the supervision of a remedial gymnast (or physiotherapist), there are certain simple tests of function suitable for the consulting room that have been found useful as quick tests of recovery of function for the major peripheral joints:

(1) Ankle: Squat jump – the patient does a full

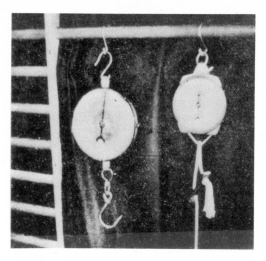

Fig 2 *Types of spring balance used in measuring the single spring lift*

knees bend and then jumps as high as he can from this position, landing on tiptoe; if he can do this with equal distribution of weight and without pain, the ankle should stand up to most sporting activities.

(2) Knee: Full squat and bounce – the patient goes into a full squat and then bounces at the end of this movement, forcibly flexing the knee with his body weight; if this can be done through a full range and without pain, the knee is unlikely to have any significant residual disability.

(3) Hip: Hopping on injured leg – the hip-joint, is, of course, rarely injured apart from dislocation or muscle injury surrounding the joint; in the former, if the patient can jump on the affected leg without pain, functional recovery can be judged as being satisfactory.

(4) Shoulder: Rotation in abduction – with the shoulder abducted to a right angle, the elbow flexed to a right angle and the forearm in a neutral position, full external and then full internal rotation are attempted and compared to the opposite side; this indicates whether the range is full and also, in the case of a rotator cuff lesion, that the healing is complete, as otherwise pain is felt on this manœuvre because of the impingement of still inflamed soft tissues between the acromion and the greater tuberosity of the humerus.

(5) Elbow: Press up – to do a full press up with

155

equal distribution of weight on the two sides requires a full range of movement of the elbow without pain.

(6) Wrist: Forced dorsiflexion – if a patient can lean his body weight on the fully dorsiflexed wrist without pain, there is unlikely to be any significant residual disability.

Finally there is the really detailed assessment of function as done in the gymnasium by the remedial gymnast (or physiotherapist). Many remedial gymnasts now use circuit training in their rehabilitation programmes and each circuit training is obviously designed for the type of case that is being dealt with. Thus the circuit training used in the rehabilitation of an injured coalminer would be different from that used in the rehabilitation of an injured athlete, and even in the case of the athlete it would vary according to his particular sport.

As an example, I describe below the circuit training devised by my remedial gymnast, Mr M Clement, at The Durham Miners Rehabilitation Centre at Chester-le-Street, for the final stages of rehabilitation of a Rugby player with a cruciate ligament injury of the knee, which had to be surgically repaired. It was felt that by the time the patient could do all these tests of function without difficulty and at a good speed, he was undoubtedly ready to return to Rugby training under the supervision of his coach.

The circuit used lasted for fifteen minutes and consisted of eight activities of one and a half minutes each:

First activity – Three half-minute periods of hop skipping.
Second activity – Fifty step ups on the injured leg.
Third activity – Balanced walking on balance and exercise bench placed upside down.
Fourth activity – Static cycling covering approximately one mile.
Fifth activity – Walking up and down an incline on balance and exercise bench at an angle of 45 degrees to give a 1 in 1 gradient.
Sixth activity – Three sets of squats thirty times each.
Seventh activity – Quadriceps power training: the patient does five series of 5 RM lifts, holding full extension for five seconds on each lift.
Eighth activity – Short sprints 10 seconds sprinting, 10 seconds walking.

Circuit training is useful not only for purposes of assessment, but also in the rehabilitation of all types of injury. It must be devised to suit not only the needs of the particular injury, but also

156

of the particular sport or occupation of the patient.

In summary, it is important to stress that in the case of sportsmen, particularly of national or international status, it is essential for the physician or surgeon treating the case and supervising the rehabilitation programme to liaise with the coach from an early stage, not only so that the doctor can fully understand the stresses involved in the sport concerned, but also because the coach can help in the planning of the circuit training used in reconditioning the patient. This sort of liaison already occurs with advantage between hospital doctors and industrial medical officers and between hospital doctors and disablement resettlement officers of the Department of Employment and Productivity.

REFERENCES
DeLorme T L (1945) *J. Bone Jt Surg.* **27,** 645
Zinovieff A (1951) *Brit. J. phys. Med.* **14,** 129

157

Late Effects of Neglected Soft Tissue Injury

Dr Hugh C Burry

Neglect of an injury may be the responsibility of the patient or of the doctor. On the one hand, the player may regard his symptoms as trivial in the early stages, as he often does with lesions of the adductor origin, or may, in his anxiety to return to training before his hard-won fitness is lost, disregard his doctor's advice. On the other hand, the advice he receives may be poor – ill-informed, unenthusiastic or, not uncommonly, both. This paper examines some of the consequences of the neglect of soft tissue injuries and, in doing so, regards mistreatment and nontreatment as one and the same thing.

A tear of a muscle, whether it be the result of intrinsic strain or external force, results in rupture of muscle fibres, interstitial tissue, muscle sheath and, most important, blood vessels. Within a few hours the resultant extravasated blood will have clotted and as retraction takes place, the plasma is squeezed out and rapidly absorbed. Left behind are the fibrous clot and the formed elements. The body's response consists of: (1) The activation of plasminogen to plasmin which promotes fibrinolysis. (2) The arrival of phagocytes to digest and ingest the necrotic muscle and blood cells. (3) Endothelial budding, producing a maze of new capillaries which invade the clot and speed resorption. (4) The proliferation of fibroblasts which lay down new collagen in the framework of the fibrin reticulum to produce scarring.

The factors which influence rate of healing are: (1) Age and physical fitness. (2) Nutrition – especially vitamin C. (3) Endocrine status – particularly steroids. (4) Blood supply to the part. (5) Presence of infection. (6) Mobility – as in bones. (7) Amount of tissue destruction.

It is the doctor's responsibility to ensure that the most favourable conditions are obtained. Thus, he must be certain that every effort is made to improve circulation, to see that nutrition is adequate, and to provide immobility where this is indicated.

The effects of this healing process, if unguided by rational therapy, are not all favourable. Sound healing may occur, but chronic granulations producing only weak collagenous fibres may fail to produce sound healing. On the other hand, vigorous scarring may produce adhesions to neighbouring structures. If the hæmatoma was large, a large mass of granulations leading ultimately to dense fibrosis – the organized hæmatoma – may result. One of the properties of young collagenous fibres is to contract with ageing, and in neglected cases this may result in shortening of the muscle. Finally, the hæmatoma may be invaded by osteoblasts, leading to the condition of myositis ossificans.

It is not always appreciated that lesions of muscles occur in three separate settings and that these require quite different management. If the lesion consists of an avulsion of the origin, characterized clinically by a diffuse brawny swelling of the muscle, initial rest is indicated to avoid the possibility of further bleeding or, worse, the complication of myositis ossificans. If the lesion is a partial avulsion of the tendinous insertion or origin of the muscle, as is common in the adductor longus, the poverty of blood supply dictates that complete rest should be prescribed to avoid the weak granulations that predispose to recurrent injury and chronic pain. Conversely, where the lesion is in the belly of the muscle, early activity is essential.

The first opportunity for neglect occurs immediately after the injury. The man who, after spraining a joint or tearing a muscle, has no pressure dressing applied and instead of going home and elevating the part, retires to the bar to take in a few pints of the world's greatest analgesic, will undoubtedly have a much greater hæmatoma and consequently a much slower convalescence.

Extravasation of large amounts of blood is the first fruit of neglect. The other ill effects follow as healing proceeds.

Contusions of the quadriceps muscle are common, especially in the body contact sports, and it is not uncommon, two weeks after injury, to find a large mass of firm, tender fibrous tissue in the substance of the muscle. This organized hæmatoma has the effect of: (1) Limiting stretch of the muscle, partly by its own resistance to stretch and partly by causing a pain-induced reflex spasm. (2) Causing adhesions to other parts of the quadriceps, so interfering with the normal gliding. (3) Limiting activity, causing loss of muscle bulk and strength, leading to: (4) Instability of the knee and possible damage to articular cartilage.

Weeks of treatment may be required to repair this damage. Shortwave diathermy or ultrasonics, together with deep massage, will break up the mass and allow a freer range of movement. The muscle should be built up by resisted exercises and light training resumed as soon as the knee becomes completely stable. Infiltration with steroid and local anæsthetic will also help at this stage.

Occasionally, the hæmatoma may become a wall of organization clot containing a pool of serum. Apart from disturbing the function of the muscle, this cyst is an ideal situation for infection to flourish. Infection may be introduced by well-intentioned attempts to evacuate the cyst and is even more vigorous if at the same time corticosteroid has been injected. Infection may also result from a transient bacteræmia, and uncontrollable infection with resistant anaerobic streptococci has been known to terminate fatally.

Myositis ossificans is the result of an invasion of the hæmatoma by osteoblasts. Whether these come from a damaged periosteum or are the result of differentiation of multipotent mesenchymal cells is unknown. Against the former theory is the fact that there sometimes appears to be a gap between the periosteum and the new bone, but this may be due to the particular chemical conditions necessary for bone to be deposited. Since the condition almost always follows avulsion of muscle from bone, as in the quadriceps or brachialis when the elbow is dislocated, it is on the whole more likely that the osteoblasts have a periosteal origin. It appears to be more common following repeated trauma, which may take the form of too vigorous active exercises or enthusiastic passive exercise with forcible stretching.

Once myositis ossificans has started, the part must be rested and therapy restricted to shortwave diathermy and gentle static contractions until decrease of pain and heat indicates that activity has subsided. Normal function then returns surprisingly quickly and the training schedule can be stepped up rapidly.

Tears of the hamstrings cause disability apparently out of proportion to the severity of the damage. In the absence of proper management there is a very real risk of recurrent tears. The lesion usually occurs in the belly of the muscle and improper management will result in a palpable mass in the posterior thigh with limitation of straight leg raising and pain on running, felt just as the affected leg swings through. This pain and restriction of range of movement is in part due to shortening of the muscle and in part to adhesions to surrounding structures, inhibiting free movement of the muscle sheath.

If rest is prescribed during the healing phase, shortening of the muscle is likely to take place as the collagen shrinks. If hamstring tears tend to occur in individuals with a comparative shortness of this muscle, the likelihood of relapses when training is resumed is great – the more so since the scar forms an inelastic segment, and like a cane flyrod with a rigid ferrule, the failure tends to occur adjacent to the unyielding part. This can be avoided by starting active exercises, within the scope allowed by pain, no more than forty-eight hours after the accident.

Faced with the established results of neglect, the treatment will consist of local corticosteroid injections together with deep massage and active and passive mobilizing exercises. Training may be resumed at slowly increasing speeds and considerable reassurance will be required to persuade the athlete that any pain that he experiences is not of sinister significance.

Avulsions of a tendinous origin are most commonly seen in adductor longus, and in the common extensor origin from the lateral epicondyle. Here the key to successful management is to order complete rest with periodic careful controlled stretching from the outset. The problem is that the symptoms are commonly relatively trivial at the outset and the athlete with an adductor tendinitis finds that the pain and stiffness wear off after a short period of activity. Later the pain becomes more intractable but by this time granulations have formed. At this stage rest allows a weak attachment to take place, but a return to activity soon breaks this down. Sound repair can only take place if an injection of corticosteroid into the site of maximum tenderness is combined with complete rest and careful stretching of the affected muscle. In extremely resistant cases, tenotomy is performed. As the duration of inactivity may be more than a month, depending on the degree of chronicity of the lesion, the price in terms of loss of fitness that the athlete pays for the initial error is exorbitant.

A similar lesion is lateral epicondylitis, commonly known as 'tennis elbow'. Here inflammatory changes in the injured common extensor tendon may spread to the capsule of the radiohumeral joint causing pain on supination of the forearm as well as pain on extension of the wrist and fingers. In some cases, calcification may occur. Management is similar to that of the adductor lesion – steroid injections, rest and tenotomy if nothing else works.

Taking avulsion a step further, a flake of bone may separate with the tendon, as occurs quite commonly with the digital extensor tendons.

If this lesion is not treated by immediate immobilization, or possibly surgical reconstruction, the condition of 'mallet finger' results. Finally, avulsion may include an epiphysis, as appears to be the case at the insertion of the patellar tendon into the tibial tubercle in Osgood-Schlatter disease.

Occasionally, when the ankle is dorsiflexed and inverted suddenly, the peroneal retinaculum may be ruptured, allowing the peroneal tendons to dislocate forwards over the fibula. If the correct diagnosis is not made, the patient develops sharp stabs of pain every time he everts his ankle due to the tendons slipping forwards, and surgical reconstruction of the retinaculum will be necessary. This might be avoided by early diagnosis and immobilization.

Achilles peritendonitis is a lesion which has ended the careers of many athletes, some of them Olympic performers. There is good reason to believe that a proportion of these cases are really degenerative conditions of the tendon causing a partial rupture which never completely heals. In fact it is surprising how often even complete rupture of the tendon is misdiagnosed. In the majority of cases, however, the pain is due to a chronic synovitis. Here, as in the adductor tendonitis, the key to successful management is a short period of complete rest with a heel raise when the pain is first noticed. If neglected at this stage, this simple lesion can become extraordinarily resistant to treatment.

Further problems may arise if corticosteroid injections are employed, particularly into the tendon itself. The blood supply of the tendon is so tenuous that the increase in pressure resulting from the injection may effectively cut it off, leading to necrosis and subsequent rupture.

Finally, the most important result of neglected injury for the athlete is loss of fitness. An Olympic medal-winning rowing crew were assessed prior to starting training, again nine months later, at the time of the Olympics, and finally one month after the Games. In the latter period they had done no training at all. It was found that in a four-week period they had regressed to their basal condition.

Obviously it is the duty of the medical adviser to return his patient to training as soon as possible and the loss of fitness that results from his failure to do so is the most important effect of mistreatment.

It is the view of many doctors that athletic injuries are trivialities, that athletes are very lucky to be so fit and that they should accept a prolonged period of rest without any other treatment and not waste the doctor's time. Such a view is not only damaging to the standing of the medical profession but totally irresponsible.

160

Medical Aspects of Skiing*

MERRITT H. STILES, M.D.

INTRODUCTION

While most health factors related to skiing are orthopedic or surgical, there are a few which might be considered primarily medical. They will be considered under
five headings, frostbite, heart attacks, public health, medical contraindications to skiing, and skiing as a therapeutic tool.

FROSTBITE

Frostbite can be a serious problem, though rarely so for
Alpine skiers. Colorado as a state has had a rather high
incidence of frostbite; the University of Colorado Medical
Center, for example, having had more than 100 admissions in a ten-year period, with almost 100 amputations.[1]
Most of the admissions were either alcoholics sleeping it
off in a snowbank, or were the results of automobile accidents in the high mountains. There were five mountain
climbers who became stranded, and two who were lost on
a ski touring expedition. Inadequate clothing in the alco-
holic and automobile accident groups was an important
factor.

Cold weather studies, in the Antarctic for example,
have lead to the belief that the most effective insulation
against chilling is a layer of warm air, such as is afforded
by Scandinavian fishnet type underwear, with about an
inch between weaves, and covered by a closely woven

*Presented February 1, 1971, Conference on Skiing Injuries,
American Academy of Orthopedic Surgeons, Snowmass-at-
Aspen, Colorado.

shirt such as cotton twill rather than by loosely woven wool. A light sweater and an impervious parka serve as outer garments. Such a combination provides much more effective protection than does some of the heavy, bulky clothing. Clothing that fits too tightly eliminates this layer of warm air, and shoes that fit too snugly increase the possibility of cold injury.

Protection of the head is also important, with a parka type hood rather than a cap with ear flaps. A nylon pile type of hood is better than fur, which tends to accumulate ice crystals.

It is of interest that observations in Korea demonstrated that persons who grew up in a mountainous or other cold weather environment were less susceptible to cold injury than were Southerners, whether white or black. This observation was duplicated in experimental studies, when rabbits raised in outside hutches in cold weather, with low ambient temperature, proved less susceptible to cold injury than did rabbits raised during warm weather. In the now famous Pro Football Championship game held at Green Bay, Wisconsin in weather well below zero, the incidence cold injury, among the Dallas squad was several times that of the "boys" from Green Bay. It was not clear whether the increased resistance of cold-reared humans and animals was the result of some type of cellular adaptation, the result of an improved knowledge of how to protect one's self, or the result of some combination of both factors.

From the standpoint of the Alpine skier, the most common cold injury is superficial frostbite, or frostnip as it is often called. This develops principally in the exposed face, the cheeks, chin or tip of the nose. It is not apt to occur unless the temperature falls near the zero Fahrenheit range. The chill factor brought on by rapid air motion, as with fast skiing or wind, increases the likelihood of cold injury. After an initial period of discomfort, often unnoticed, the tissues involved become white and sensation-less. Treatment is simple, warming the frozen area as rapidly as possible. Cupping a hand over the frozen area, or burying a frozen nose tip in a companion's axilla, may be effective emergency treatment. It is probably best, when possible, to go indoors.

The frostnip victim is usually unaware that he has gotten into trouble; it is particularly important not to ski alone in very cold weather since recognition of cold injury by a companion will lead to prompt treatment and avoidance of prolonged freezing with more serious tissue injury. If treatment is prompt, there are usually no after effects other than a little superficial blistering, and possibly a local increased sensitivity to cold for a period of time.

While frostbite of the extremities would seem to be a likely development, it is rarely encountered in Alpine skiing, other than in the devoutly careless or reckless skier who ignores the rules of ski safety and becomes lost for a prolonged period. The discomfort of cold hands and feet, and the interference with effective skiing, will usually send the skier indoors before frostbite has a chance to develop.

The most effective treatment for frostbite is of course prevention. Concentrating on lodge skiing if the temperature is below zero, particularly if there is a strong wind, is completely effective. The avid skier is not apt to stay indoors just because the weather is too cold, however, but he may protect his face by wearing a knitted mask with eyeholes and with an opening for the mouth and nostrils. The leather facial masks recently available presumably eliminate some of the discomforts of the knitted masks, and a vinyl-covered foam rubber thermoshield to cover both the face and neck is available and effective.

Too frequent and too thorough bathing has been considered to increase the likelihood of frostbite, through the removal of protective skin oils. While this is of little consequence in Alpine skiing, it has been suggested that the use of preshave and after shave lotions might increase the risk of facial frostnip, though it should be pointed out that females are not immune. The use of protective facial creams has been suggested, but their usefulness has not been demonstrated.

HEART ATTACKS

The heart attacks which on rare occasions develop on ski slopes give us another reason to be thankful that our ski slopes are patrolled by the volunteer members of the National Ski Patrol System, or in larger resort-type areas, by professional patrols. Prompt removal by toboggan to the emergency room, and subsequent prompt transfer to a hospital, minimize unfavorable complications. Many ski areas now have physicians available, able to supply emergency treatment even before hospital transfer.

While sudden death has been reported all too frequently in joggers, I have not encountered any report of such a death in a skier, though it seems probable that a few might have occurred. The reasons for the difference in incidence of sudden death in jogging and in skiing are not clear, though a possible factor could be the difference in energy output. In jogging and running energy expendi-

163

ture is continuous and high, often 75 percent of maximum, or more, leading to exhaustion in a short period of time. In downhill skiing, on the other hand, energy expenditure is at a much lower level, usually not more than 25 to 40 percent of maximum, and there are frequent interruptions to rest, to converse, to view the scenery, to adjust equipment, or to ride a lift in preparation for another run.

Another possible factor is the relative state of preparatory conditioning. Most skiers make at least a modest effort to get in shape before the ski season, and perhaps carry over some degree of conditioning, as well as of skill, from the previous season. Many of the jogging deaths have apparently occurred in individuals who have gone precipitately from a life of physical inactivity to one of strenuous exertion. By way of contrast, the only skiers involved in energy expenditure comparable to that of running, cross country ski competition, have gone through prolonged conditioning and training programs.

Public Health Aspects

While acute pulmonary edema is clearly a medical problem, it is altitude-related, and will be discussed in another paper. There are other respiratory problems, however, which develop whenever large numbers of skiers and spectators congregate, as during the F I S World Championships, or during the Winter Olympic Games, problems similar to those which develop anytime large numbers of persons gather in areas with limited sanitary facilities, modified somewhat by winter temperatures. Dr. William W. Stiles, Professor of Public Health at the University of California at Berkeley and Medical Director for the VIIIth Winter Olympic Games as Squaw Valley, reported that 2200 names were recorded in their sickbook during the Games.[2] About 200 were spectators, 50 were athletes (this is not a realistic reflection of the actual incidence of injury or illness among the athletes, since most of the larger teams had their own physicians), another 50 were officials, and the remaining 1900 were Service personnel. Approximately half of those listed had surgical problems; the medical problems were those of infection or communicable disease. The common cold and influenza were frequent. There were only 42 cases of gastroenteritis, thanks to the rigid control of food-handling and dishwashing techniques, and of water supply and sewage disposal. The incidence of influenza in the Winter Games was significantly lower than during the pre-Olympic Games in 1959. It was felt that the impor-

164

tant factors were the earlier peaking of the 1960 epidemic, the extra precautions to segregate contestants and team officials from other personnel, and improvements in sanitation of food, air and drink, rather than the prophylactic immunization given some 490 persons. Of this group, 57 became ill for an attack rate of 7.6 percent, quite similar to that of a group who received only placebos.

MEDICAL CONTRAINDICATIONS TO SKIING

Since skiing is possible at a wide range of energy expenditures, there are few absolute medical contraindications. Any person who can walk could at least undertake cross-country skiing. A greater degree of physical agility would be desirable, of course, for downhill skiing. Any severe illness, particularly if recent, would be a contraindication, as it would be for any physical activity requiring a significant expenditure of energy. Parkinsonism, unless minimal, and hemiplegia, unless there has been essentially complete recovery, would be definite contraindications because of interference with the exact control and timing demanded in skiing. Compensated heart disease, on the other hand, would ordinarily not be a contraindication to recreational skiing.

SKIING AS A THERAPEUTIC TOOL

To some physicians, the most important health aspect of skiing is its usefulness as a therapeutic tool. The most serious health problem of the present generation is coronary heart disease, now the most frequent cause of death in the American male, and still increasing gradually in incidence. Many studies have been made on the factors involved in its development, the role of cholesterol and other fatty substances in coronary arteriosclerosis, a factor underlying most heart attacks, is now almost as well known to the layman as to the scientist. The layman is generally not so familiar, however, with the studies which have related coronary heart disease to physical inactivity.

One of the early studies was on the comparative incidence of heart attacks in London bus drivers and conductors. The drivers, whose days were almost entirely sedentary, had many more attacks than did the conductors, who kept busy running up and down the steps to the upper deck.

Other studies have shown similar results. Review of records of the Health Insurance Plan of New York revealed heart attacks were less frequent in physically active persons than in those who led sedentary lives. If an attack did occur in the physically active group, it was much less likely to be fatal, and recovery was more rapid.

An interesting and thought-provoking study was made on a group of Irishmen living in or near Boston, and on a comparable group of their brothers and cousins still living in Ireland. Though those in Ireland ate more than did their American relatives, their weight averaged 10 pounds less, and the incidence of coronary heart disease was much lower. The most significant difference between the two groups, from the standpoint of possible causative factors, was the greater degree of physical activity in those living in Ireland, and it was concluded that this was the major factor in the lower heart disease incidence.

With the relationship noted between physical inactivity and coronary heart disease, it was not surprising that exercise programs were developed for use in the recovery phases following heart attacks. The reports on such programs, and reports on preventive programs, have been almost universally favorable. Controlled, graduated exercise has even been shown to be of benefit in angina pectoris, where physical activity generally induces cardiac pain.

Why does exercise help the heart? Unfortunately, the answer still must be "We really don't know, though we do have some ideas." Under some conditions, vigorous exercise increases the size of collateral coronary vessels. Observations on veteran handball players, whose hearts functioned effectively in spite of definite evidence of damage to significant areas of heart muscle, suggest that this may be a factor in some individuals. Another thought-provoking suggestion is that physical inactivity sensitizes the heart muscle to the damaging effects of stress-produced catecholamines. Wilhelm Raab, of the University of Vermont, has stated that an important factor in cardiac susceptibility is "the widespread deficiency of antiadrenergic counter regulation that results from habitual lack of physical exercise."

The beneficial effects of exercise are not confined to the heart. The improved feeling of well-being from regular active exercise has long been known. And exercise is being increasingly recognized as an important factor in weight control; many overweight individuals do very poorly on food restriction alone, but will lose steadily if adequate exercise is combined with an appropriate, and usually less rigid, restriction of the food intake. It is distressing, with knowledge of this sort available, that the modern male should have succumbed so completely to the allure of labor-saving, and exercise-sparing, devices. It has been said, and only semi-facetiously, that the invention of the automobile did more damage to the American male heart than any other single factor.

More and more physicians feel that active exercise is a must if an individual is to remain in optimum health, and live life to the fullest; such physicians tend to prescribe an exercise program, in addition to whatever other therapeutic measures may be indicated, when the average, flabby American male appears as a patient.

What type of exercise? The profession seems to be approaching general agreement that the most important forms of exercise are those which stress the heart and lungs. Most forms of calisthenics, and many types of gymnasium activity, are primarily muscle building, and besides being boring, do little if anything for the cardiopulmonary system, which is most benefited when the body's largest muscle masses, the legs, are used vigorously. Walking, hiking, climbing stairs, are good preparatory exercises, but are not vigorous enough for maximum benefit. Once the health-seeker has gotten into reasonable condition, he should advance gradually to more vigorous activities. Skipping rope and in place running are excellent, but the scenery doesn't change much. Jogging and running outdoors have more to offer, though complications may arise in settled neighborhoods. A secluded lakeshore road, though at times dusty, rocky and hilly, may be more attractive. And even more attractive might be Per-Olaf Astrand's Swedish course, finishing with a sauna and an icy dip.[3]

Where does skiing fit in? It provides vigorous exercise of a truly beneficial type. It is sustained enough so that it may be an important factor in weight control. Even more important, it is fun. Once its joys have ensnared him, the weary and often discouraging hours of instruction and practice seem but unimportant steps on the skier's way to competence, and he happily turns to such substitute summer activities as jogging, swimming, cycling or mountain climbing, just to be in top condition when the first snowflakes fall.

REFERENCES

1. Weatherly-White, R-C-A.: Prevention of Frostbite in Winter Sports, p 231-246, Proceedings, Conference on Winter Sports Injuries, State Medical Society of Wisconsin, 330 E. Lakeside St., Madison, Wisconsin, 1970.
2. Stiles, W. W.: Prevention of Infection and Communicable Disease in Ski Areas, p 283-291, Ibid.
3. Astrand, P.-O.: Concluding Remarks, p 907-911, Proceedings of the International Symposium on Physical Activity and Cardiovascular Health, Canad. Med. Assoc. Jovr. 96, (Mar. 25) 1967.

E. C. PERCY, M.D., F.R.C.S.(C), F.A.C.S.
Montreal, Quebec

THE SNOWMOBILE: FRIEND OR FOE?

The first snowmobiling vehicle was built in 1923 in Valcourt, Quebec, by Joseph-Armand Bombardier, at the time only 16 years of age. It consisted of a set of sleigh runners propeller-driven by a four-cylinder Ford Model T engine. A few years later Bombardier produced the first motorized wheel-driven treated vehicle. This model was made by mounting a cabin on a car chassis powered by an automobile engine. Bombardier's interest in snow vehicles continued, and in 1936 he developed patents on his newly-designed track, suspension system, and sprocket. With the development of a proper propelling system, he started producing and selling these vehicles. Over the next decade, which included the war years, production increased, including school buses, ambulances, snowploughs, and even armored troop carriers. In 1958 Bombardier produced the prototype of the first personal snowmobile, and the following year 225 of these machines were sold. The intrepid inventor died in 1964, too soon to see the impact his snowmobile was to make on North America over the ensuing years.

It has been estimated that between 600,000 and 650,000 of these vehicles will be sold in the snowbelt area of Canada and the U.S.A. (19 states) in the 1971–72 winter season. This should bring the total number of snowmobiles in this region to well over 2 million units by the spring of 1972. There are at present some 86 companies in Canada, U.S.A., Europe, and Asia producing these vehicles for marketing in North America. The machines vary in price from $700 to $1,800, and weigh from 250 to 600 lb. Their internal combustion engines are capable of developing 10 to 50 horsepower, enabling the driver to race through the snow at top speeds ranging from 35 to 100 mph.

There can be little doubt as to the value of these tracked vehicles in the snowbelt region. They have become a way of life, and contribute a great deal towards solving man's main preoccupation of finding a pleasant way of spending his increased leisure time. It is a recreational activity which is fast displacing some of the more common social activities. Indeed, there are now many thousands of snowmobile clubs in North America. People living in the rural areas are no longer confined to the house during a large part of the winter, but can get out and not only visit with their neighbors but also travel around the great outdoors with these same neighbors. The snowmobile's important role in mercy missions during severe snowstorms cannot be overemphasized. The vehicle is, of course, indispensable in the Arctic, and has now almost entirely replaced travel by dogsled. Injuries and fatalities are at a minimum amongst the Eskimos, due to the absence of highways and railways in the Arctic.

Associated with this increased role of the snowmobile in our society, there has developed a growing concern by the public at large and the medical profession. The former is concerned with the threat to the environment, the latter about the alarming increase in severe injuries and fatalities.

Those concerned with ecology are aroused about the danger these vehicles pose to wildlife and trees. The noise factor, of course, is real, as indeed is air pollution due to this increased usage of the internal combustion engine. The country cottage, which was once inaccessible in winter, is now no longer safe from break-ins, and insurance rates will be affected accordingly. Probably the damage to small trees has been over-emphasized, but certainly wild animals and birds will be driven further away into the hinterlands. Whereas formerly the professional hunter could possibly cover a trap-line of only 6 to 10 miles on skis or snowshoes, he can now lay traps along a 50- or even a 100-mile trap-line to ensure a larger catch.

The medical profession are understandably concerned about the increasing carnage on the snow ways, highways, and even railways. In 1970, 118 deaths were reported in Canada as the direct result of snowmobile accidents, and 82 lives were lost in the U.S.A. during the same period. Satisfactory statistics are not readily available as to the total number of injuries sustained by the 1.6 million snowmobile users in our North American snowbelt in 1970. Several studies over the past few years are, however,

168

worthy of mention. Chism and Soule (1) reported a series of 103 patients injured in snowmobile accidents in 1969. In this group 37 patients sustained injuries to the lower extremities, the most common area involved. There were also 15 cases of vertebral compression fractures in the series, many of which were multiple. This latter injury is, of course, the direct result of bouncing on the hard seats over large bumps or jumps, or of being ejected from the machine. Martyn (4) analyzed hospitalized snowmobile injuries over a 3-year period and reported on 135 cases. As might be expected, the area most commonly involved was the lower extremity (50% of the cases). The larger percentage were males with an age spread from 2 to 63 years. Perhaps the most serious nonfatal injury is that of the "wishbone injury" discussed by Erskine (3) in an editorial in this *Journal* in 1970. This frightful injury results when the projecting knee is trapped in passing close to a stationary object while the opposite knee is held by the seat of the snowmobile. The unfortunate victim is literally torn asunder by this injury. Withington and Hall (5) report on a questionnaire study of 59 injuries in a 1-year period. Collisions between the machine and fixed objects, other motion vehicles, other snowmobiles, and—even more important—other people, accounted for 21 of these injuries. These latter injuries occurred among pedestrians as well as passengers, due to the patient's falling out of a machine and being hit by another vehicle following behind. Again, the larger number of injuries were amongst males, the age range being from 8 to 68 years. E. B. Hendrick, in a presentation on injuries associated with winter sports, discussed head injuries associated with snow vehicles (unpublished data). He reported injuries to the head from passengers ejected not only from the prime vehicle but also from the trailer. He also mentioned scalping injuries from the continuously turning tread in an overturned vehicle.

J. J. Wiley and D. H. Johnson (unpublished data) reported on a clinical survey of 161 patients treated in the Ottawa area during the 1970–71 season. In their series, 23% of the injured snowmobilers were hospitalized. As in all other reported series, the lower extremity was the most commonly involved, and 47% of this group were treated for injuries to this region. They found that the commonest mechanism of injury was ejection, followed closely by collision and then machine failure. The time of accident was equally divided between daytime and nightime misadventure. These authors concluded that the major portion of the blame must rest with the driver. They stressed the role of driver education and legislation to reduce the accident rate.

The most recent medical article on snowmobile injuries has been contributed by Daniel and Midgley (2). The authors present four severe facial injuries which resulted from accidents in which the driver was wearing the generally accepted crash helmet. They feel that the incidence and severity of facial injuries could be reduced by incorporating a contoured face bar into this standard helmet.

Indirect injuries can, of course, result from snowmobiling. Acute myocardial infarction is not uncommon, for example, from the stress of lifting the machine back on the trail or having to walk out of the bush through deep snow because of a faulty engine or an empty gas tank. Mention should also be made of the "wind-chill" factor resulting in the freezing of exposed parts of the body when travelling at high speeds. At a temperature of zero F and a speed of 30 mph, the equivalent temperature the skin is exposed to is −48 F!

The vast majority, if not all deaths, are of course avoidable or preventable. In Quebec last year, 63 deaths were reported. Thirty-six of these occurred on the road where the machines are legally banned except for designated crossing points. In 1969, 93 deaths were attributed to snowmobile accidents in Canada. This figure climbed to 118 in 1970, an increase of 26.9%. How did the victims die? Collisions with other vehicles accounted for 55.3%; 11.6% were due to snowmobiles crashing through ice or running into open stretches of water; 1.8% were thrown off their vehicles; 5.3% had collisions with pedestrians; 3.6% ran their vehicles into fences or cables; 8.9% struck other hidden objects; 1.8% collided with trains; and finally in 11.7% death resulted from heart attacks or freezing to death.

From the foregoing rather gloomy statistics, one would assume that this vehicle is a rather dangerous machine. This assumption would be correct with the present unrestricted use of these machines and in the absence of legislation. That the driver rather than the machine is at fault is obvious. At present, generally speaking, anyone of any age can drive these machines. There are no mandatory screening tests for skill, training, experience, or medical status of the driver. Add to this the use of alcohol on a cold night drive, and one can readily appreciate why most accidents occur at night.

Legislation is obviously essential, and should be aimed at licensing the driver after a suitable test and registration of all vehicles. The snowmobile should indeed carry a number plainly marked on each side of the machine. The machines should not be allowed within 25 yards of any road or highway, and should be allowed to cross only at designated areas. Perhaps legislation should be passed which would limit the manufacturers to two types of vehicles, a low-powered machine for general leisure use and a high-powered machine for use in organized racing areas only. A minimum age for drivers presents a problem, and most areas have legislated that only a person with a driver's license may cross a public road with a snowmobile. In Canada by early 1972, the noise level will be subject to legislation with a maximum sound intensity level of 82 decibels (a car starting off at 50 ft). Most of the snowbelt areas now prohibit hunting or carrying firearms on snow vehicles to prevent their use in tracking down virtually helpless animals in the snow. These vehicles should be barred from all wildlife preserves or national park areas. Enforcing any such legislation will, of course, require a large mobile force with adequate equipment.

The manufacturers are now sincerely trying to improve the safety features, and a good deal of work in this field is being carried out by The International Snowmobile Industry Agency. A booklet is available from the ISIA outlining the snowmobiler's code of ethics. Most manufacturers carefully outline the do's and don'ts. of safe snowmobiling in the owner's manual.

There is in the snowmobile, as in its highway counterpart the motorcycle, little if any protection between the occupant and his environment. This is, of course, an important factor in breaking down the causes of the high injury and death rate. Ideally the machine should be well balanced with a low center of gravity, and all moving parts and the engine should be covered. The steering mechanism must be made more reliable to allow for short radius turning on icy or hard surfaces. Brakes are now becoming standard features. A "dead man's throttle" should be standard equipment. All portions of the driver and the passengers should be protected so as not to project beyond the vehicle or its windshield. While unplanned dismounting might be eliminated by some sort of fixation apparatus, its use could lead to other serious injuries, or even death, by inability to dismount rapidly in an emergency situation. A roll-bar of some sort no doubt will be incorporated in the future. Finally, the use of crash helmets and goggles should be made mandatory, and although protective clothing is an expensive item, its importance should be stressed.

In summary, snowmobiling can be an enjoyable sport. It must be recognized, however, by all parties concerned—the manufacturer, the driver, and the legislation—that this vehicle is a potentially dangerous machine. It is capable of causing severe injuries and death to both occupants of the vehicle and the uninvolved bystanders, not to mention destruction to private property and a potential threat to our ecology. Sincere efforts must be made by all parties involved to ensure that the hazards of this rapidly growing leisure activity are well understood. The majority of the problems created by the snowmobile are due to "driver error," and as such are preventable.

REFERENCES

1. CHISM SE, SOULE AB: Snowmobile injuries: hazards from a popular new winter sport. *JAMA* 209:1672-1674, 1969
2. DANIEL RK, MIDGELY RD: Facial fractures in snowmobile accidents. *Plast Reconstr Surg* 49: 38-40, 1972
3. ERSKINE LA: The epidemiology of snowmobiling injuries. *J Trauma* 10:804-806, 1970
4. MARTYN JW: Snowmobile accidents. *Can Med Assoc J* 101:770-772, 1969
5. WITHINGTON RL, HALL LW: Snowmobile accidents: a review of injuries sustained in the use of snowmobiles in northern New England during 1968/1969 season. *J Trauma* 10:760-763, 1970

Skateboard Injuries in a Campus Community

STANLEY H. SCHUMAN, M.D., Dr.P.H.

Last spring, Ann Arbor and many other communities were visited by a recreational mania called "skateboarding." [1] Certain features of the sport, namely: (a) timing, and (b) extent and patterns of skateboard injury, seemed to lend themselves to an epidemiological approach.

a. *Timing of the sport* and its impact on this campus community was literally *no* accident! Many of the classic features of an acute infectious process were simulated, including an explosive "common-source"

Paper prepared for Research Symposium on Child Safety, April 21–22, 1966. University of Virginia School of Medicine (Prof. R. J. Meyer), Charlottesville, Virginia.

epidemic curve (Figs. 1, 2, 3).[5] Agent-host-environment relationships were also quite analogous:

Agent—   the profiteering dealer who sold the first 500 skateboards to sororities as spring party favors;

Hosts—   the pool of susceptibles among exam-stressed students;

Environment—the enticement of a late but balmy spring; many paved hilly slopes, glamorous advertising, and an ample supply of skateboards.

b. *Extent of injury* tended to be exaggerated or minimized by partisans, although the severity of cases seen by orthopedic surgeons was well-documented.[3] Two population surveys were made to estimate morbidity:

1. A study of admissions for falls in 21 midwestern hospitals reporting to the Professional Activity Study (PAS). There was a considerable increase in hospitalizations of youngsters for falls in 1965 compared with two preceding years in a large sample of hospitals (Fig. 4). This evidence is circumstantial because specific skateboard etiology was not coded; nonetheless, the data are impressive because of the relatively low rates of hospitalization from skateboard injury indicated from the school survey.

2. A questionnaire survey of 3,184 Ann Arbor schoolchildren, conducted in six schools in June, 1965. Although ages ranged from seven to 17 years, the emphasis was on reaching the junior high school group, whose responses to the questionnaires approached 85 per cent (Table 1). Onset of school vacation pre-

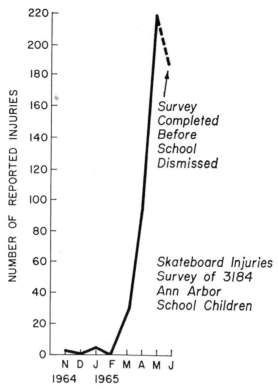

FIG. 1. Skateboard injuries survey of 3,184 Ann Arbor
school children.

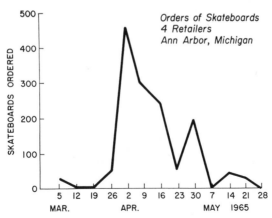

FIG. 2. Orders of skateboards, four retailers, Ann Arbor,
Michigan.

173

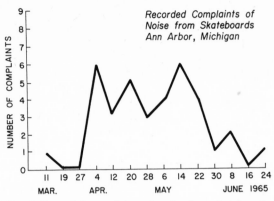

FIG. 3. Recorded complaints of noise from skateboards,
Ann Arbor, Michigan.

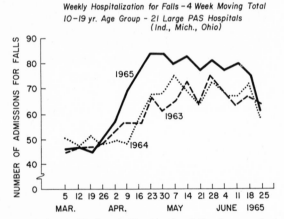

FIG. 4. Weekly hospitalization for falls—four week
moving total.

vented any serious validation of the
questionnaire; the results are presented
for *patterns* suggesting further more pre-
cise study.

It is *not* surprising that 16 of 21 fractures reported (77%) were in boys, nor
that the numbers of reported injuries
correlated very well with the number of
times skateboards were used. In contrast
to the high rate of injury (24.8%), less
than 1 per cent of skateboarders received
fractures. Only 2.7 per cent of the injuries required professional treatment.

174

Table 1. *Results of Survey of Ann Arbor Schoolchildren, June, 1965*

Age in Years	Number				Exposure: Average Person-Times	Proportion: Fractures / Injured	Proportion: Fractures / Skaters
	Respondents	Skaters	Injured	Fractures*			
9	151	93	21	1	4.9	0.05	0.01
10	192	142	32	3	5.3	0.09	0.02
11	205	151	45	4	5.4	0.09	0.03
12	190	156	43	1	5.9	0.02	0.006
13	675	570	166	5	6.0	0.03	0.01
14	550	455	82	1	5.5	0.01	0.002
15	511	417	105	4	5.7	0.04	0.01
Totals	2,474	1,984	494	19*	5.65	0.039	0.01
Per cent	100.0	80.0	24.8	0.96	—	—	—

* Two additional fractures in ages 16 and 7 not listed here. Two additional fractures in age group 11 not listed, because they occurred 24 and 48 hours after the survey, according to teachers.

175

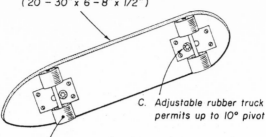

A. Platform of hard finished wood
(20 − 30" x 6 − 8" x 1/2")

C. Adjustable rubber truck
permits up to 10° pivot

B. Ball-bearinged wheels − mounted in pairs
(metal, rubber, plastic)

FIG. 5. Skateboard.

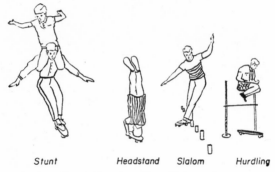

| Stunt | Headstand | Slalom | Hurdling |

FIG. 6. Skateboarding, illustrated.

Although small numbers limit the value of age-specific rates, it is evident from Table 1 that seven of 19 fractures occurred in the age groups ten and 11; thus 37 per cent of the fractures occurred in 15 per cent of the skateboarders. It is noteworthy that in another series of 33 skateboard fractures reported from another campus community, the two most severe fractures were in a boy aged 11 (skull fracture) and a boy aged 12 (compound fracture).[1]

These data suggest that, even within a relatively narrow age group (9–15 years), the hazards of skateboarding may *not* be equally distributed. As is well known, a year or two difference in chronologic age can make a sig-

176

nificant difference in coordination and margins of safety.[4] Risk-taking behavior, cheaper and inferior equipment, and other factors may contribute to injuries being more severe in ten- to 12-year-old boys than in those a little older.

Acknowledgment

The above data could not have been collected without the cooperation of the Ann Arbor School District, the University School, the Parochial Schools of Ann Arbor, and the Commission on Professional and Hospital Activities (P.A.S.).

References

1. Kincaid, C. K.: The high price of skateboarding. Quart. Bull., Wisc. State Board of Health 17: 9, 1965.
2. Life Magazine, May 14, 1965, Cover and pp. 126–134. Skateboards—The craze, the menace.
3. Liver, J. A. and Wiley, J. J.: Skurfing injuries. Canad. Med. Assn. J. 93: 651, 1965.
4. Pierson, W. R. and Montoye, H. J.: Movement time, reaction time, and age. J. Geront. 13: 418, 1958.
5. Slee, V. N., Perlman, J. M., Schuman, S. H. and Leighton, E.: The potential of P.A.S. for epidemiologic research, read before the Epidemiology Section of the A.P.H.A. in Chicago, October, 1965.

Mountain Accidents

N. F. KIRKMAN.

M. K. HARTLEY.

SIR,—Details of mountain accidents for 1967 are given in the Tables. The figures are based on accident report forms returned from official mountain rescue posts to the Mountain Rescue Committee. There are now 65 official mountain rescue posts ; they are situated in all the mountainous areas of Great Britain. In all cases the victim sustained physical injury, but in addition to the accidents recorded many searches and rescues were undertaken for persons lost, cragfast, or trapped in caves ; also 200 cases of injury to skiers were reported for the year, chiefly in Scotland.

There has been a slight increase in the total number of mountain accidents in 1967 compared with 1964 and 1965.[1] However, there were slightly more accidents in 1966 than 1967. This pause in the steady increase in the number of accidents each year was probably due to the widespread epidemic of foot-and-mouth disease in the last quarter of 1967. During this time the number of walkers and climbers was greatly reduced by voluntary co-operation of walkers, ramblers, and climbers with the farmers and agricultural authorities.

Table I shows that roughly one quarter of accidents have occurred in each of the three main climbing areas—Wales, the Lake District, and Scotland—with the Pennines and sea cliffs making up the remaining quarter. The accident incidence in the various hilly districts remains practically constant. Table I also shows that again the proportion of accidents between walkers, climbers, and cavers remains constant when compared with previous figures.[1] It will be seen that there are a few more walkers than climbers involved in accidents.

TABLE II.—*Nature of Injury*

Head and back including fractures ...	54
Fractured limbs	82
Heart attack	1
Exposure and frostbite	18
Found dead	3
Drowned	13

Injuries to the lower limb and head are the most common type of injury encountered. The wearing of a firm protective helmet (similar to the industrial helmet) by climbers is increasing, but the fashion is not yet sufficiently established to reduce the number of head injuries.

Inflatable " jet " splints have been used with satisfaction in the first-aid management of fractures of the lower limb.[2][3] Inflatable splints have only been issued to selected and experienced mountain rescue teams. Instructions have been given to users to keep the pressure in the splint at a minimum consistent with the immobilization of the fractured limb,

TABLE I.—*Analysis of Mountain Accidents in 1967*

District	Total Accidents	Injured	Fatal	Climbing	Walking	Caving
Wales	37	34	3	16	21 (3)	—
Pennines	18	8	10	3	2	13 (10)
Scotland	50	41	9	22 (3)	28 (6)	0
Lake District	54	47	7	17 (2)	35 (5)	0
Sea cliffs, including Scotland and others ..	11	3	8	9 (7)	2 (1)	0
Totals	170	133	37	67 (12)	90 (15)	13 (10)

Figures in parentheses are fatalities and are inclusive.

to reduce the pressure in the splint every one or two hours according to the state of the patient. No report of any untoward effect has been received following the use of these splints.

Drowning accidents have increased proportionally with the increase in cliff-climbing, chiefly on the South Coast and Cornwall.

TABLE III.—*Causes of Accidents (Where Known)*

Slips	109
Belay failures	3
Climbing alone	6
Loose rock	9
Abseiling	2
Glissading	1
Bad weather	8
In caves	11
Swept into or falls into the sea ...	6

As previously reported,[1] almost half of all accidents in mountainous areas happen to young people aged 21 or less. This high incidence of youth in mountain accidents has been stressed by the Central Council for Physical Recreation, the Scottish Council for Physical Recreation, and the Mountain Rescue Committee. A mountain leadership training board has been set up by interested bodies under the aegis of the Central Council for Physical Recreation. A certificate of mountain leadership is being instituted. It is hoped that leaders of youth groups will be encouraged to take this certificate and thereby obtain a reasonable knowledge of mountaineering and suitable first aid for the hills. Cases of exposure show an increase. This may be partly due to the better recognition of the condition by rescuers owing to wider publicity in mountaineering and medical journals.[1-7]—We are, etc.,

REFERENCES

[1] Kirkman, N. F., *Brit. med. J.*, 1966, **1**, 162.
[2] Gardner, W. J., *Brit. med. J.*, 1967, **3**, 49.
[3] Gardner, W. J., *J. Amer. med. Ass.*, 1966, **196**, 491.
[4] British Mountaineering Council Publication 380, November 1964. London.
[5] Trott, O. T., *Western J. Surg.*, 1960, **68**, No. 5, p. xviii.
[6] Pugh, L. G. C. E., *Brit. med. J.*, 1967, **2**, 333.
[7] Campbell, R., *Aide Memoire Secour 1, Les Accidents dus au froid, Comité Central, Club Alpino Suisse*, 1965. Pontresina.

Mountain Accidents and Mountain Rescue in Great Britain

N. F. KIRKMAN,* M.D., F.R.C.S.

In these days of increasing leisure many more people than formerly are going to the hills for recreation and exercise. This is especially true of the young. Courses and expeditions organized by schools, climbing schools, Outward Bound schools, the Duke of Edinburgh Award Scheme, Rover and Scout groups, and other youth groups are now being held daily throughout most months of the year. In addition, the number of walking, rambling, and mountaineering clubs continues to grow. The access to mountainous areas has been made easier by the advent of the motorways and improved transport facilities. As a result of these changes the number of people visiting the Lake District, Snowdonia, the Pennines, and Scotland has probably increased tenfold in the last 20 years.

This increase in numbers has brought an increase in the number of accidents and acute illness taking place in the hills. There are now probably nearly 200 cases in England and Wales and 60 in Scotland (excluding skiing accidents) occurring annually.

Many of the public who frequent the hills and many doctors are unaware of the facilities which already exist to deal with these emergencies (*B.M.J.*, 1964).

The police are basically responsible for the care of injured persons, but they are not as a rule equipped or trained for mountain rescue, though they have rendered great help on occasions. They have been especially helpful in organizing rescues, calling out rescue teams, and assisting with transport and telecommunications. In some of the climbing centres in Wales and Scotland mountain-rescue teams have recently included a few policemen in their ranks.

Mountain-rescue Services

The problem of first aid for mountain casualties has long been recognized by the mountaineering clubs of Great Britain.

In 1936 they formed the Mountain Rescue Committee to organize mountain-rescue posts, first aid, and transport of casualties in the chief climbing centres. Since 1949 the Ministry of Health and the Home Office have recognized this committee. Authorized equipment at official mountain-rescue posts is now paid for by the National Health Service, but the costs of special equipment, climbing aids, insurance of rescuers, and clerical work are the responsibility of the Mountain Rescue Committee. On the advice of the committee and its Scottish branch new posts may be set up when the need for them has been shown to exist. The committee is now formed by representatives from the mountaineering clubs of Great Britain, other outdoor organizations—such as Youth Hostel Associations, mountain schools, the Ramblers Association—the police in Scotland, and also representatives from mountain-rescue teams.

Most of the busy mountain-rescue posts are supervised by a local mountain-rescue team. These teams are formed of volunteers, some of whom take the British Red Cross or St. John's first-aid certificates. The formation of local rescue teams has increased the efficiency of first aid and transport of the injured climbers and walkers ; some old-established teams have many notable rescues to their credit.

There are now 59 official mountain-rescue posts in Great Britain at strategic centres in mountainous areas. Their situation is shown by a blue and white plaque (Fig. 1) attached to the building where the equipment is kept. Some of the older posts are marked on the 1 in. ordnance survey map, but at times posts are moved. The exact situation of an official mountain-rescue post may be found by consulting the current edition of the *Mountain Rescue and Cave Rescue* handbook (Mountain Rescue Committee, 1965).

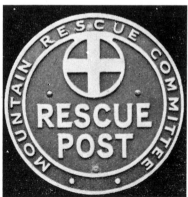

FIG. 1.—Official sign of mountain-rescue post.

Equipment of Mountain-rescue First-aid Posts

The standard equipment of official mountain-rescue first-aid posts includes a stretcher. In most posts this is a Thomas stretcher designed by Eustace Thomas, a distinguished climber and engineer. It is made from duralumin tubing, has telescopic handles, ash or laminated skids, and it is fitted with a Terylene net bed (Fig. 2). This stretcher has proved itself over many years. In Scotland the Duff and MacInnes stretchers have also been used. Both these stretchers are made in two parts which may be carried separately and united at the scene of the accident.

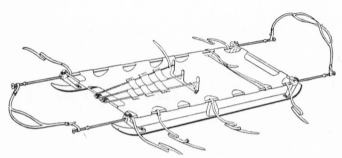

FIG. 2.—Thomas stretcher, with double Thomas splint.

Morphine (Omnopon gr. ½ in a Tubunic ampoule-syringe) is standard equipment at all official posts and its safe custody is the responsibility of the post supervisor. In all cases where morphine is used details are recorded and reported annually to the Home Office by the Issuing Officer for Morphia.

The kit, carried in two rucksacks, also includes antiseptics, bandages, arm splints, and a casualty bag. The casualty bag is a waterproofed, quilted sleeping-bag with a plastic-foam base into which the casualty is placed for transport. All official rescue kits include means of providing hot drinks, such as Thermos flasks and pressure stoves at isolated posts. Self-heating tins of soup have been most useful both for the victim and rescuers during prolonged rescues and searches.

Besides this civilian organization, the R.A.F. Mountain Rescue Service has played a great part in mountain rescue since its formation in the last war, notably in Scotland and North Wales. The units are of course superbly equipped and freely mobile and help has often been given to accident victims far from R.A.F. bases. The British Red Cross and St. John's Ambulance Brigade also maintain first-aid boxes in the Lake district and Scotland.

Mountain Accidents in 1963 and 1964

The details of mountain accidents given here have been compiled from accident reports submitted to the Mountain Rescue Committee. While more accidents may have taken place than are recorded here, the great majority of accidents occurring in the mountains of England and Wales and most of those in Scotland, excluding skiing accidents, are recorded. The type of injury and cause of the accident have been roughly classified. All official posts are given accident report forms which enable the supervisor of the post to request replacements of equipment used in the accident and to give details of the person injured and how the accident occurred. Needless to say, not all accident report forms are filled in completely, but in most cases adequate details are given (Table I).

In addition, 54 skiing accidents were reported in 1963, but probably three times as many occurred. Nine people were caught in avalanches, three being killed in the Pennines in the early part of 1963 as a result of the extraordinary snow conditions. Several climbers were injured when pitons (pegs) were pulled out during falls. In one case the falling climber dragged out four and in another he was struck on the head by his piton hammer as he fell.

Tables II and III show the nature of the injuries suffered during the two years, and, for 1964, the cause of the accidents. As far as possible the major cause of the accident is given.

More than half of the persons injured on the hills of Great Britain in 1964 were 21 or less.

TABLE II.—*Analysis of Injuries Due to Mountain Accidents in* 1963 *and* 1964

Nature of Injury	1963	1964
	%	%
Fractured limbs	33	46
Head injuries	30	24
Chest and abdominal injuries	7	7
Exposure and exhaustion	10	7
Heart failure	7	2
Miscellaneous, frostbite, drowning, unclassified	13	14

TABLE III.—*Causes of Mountain Accidents in* 1964

Cause of Accident	Number
Slips on rock and scree	60
Climbing beyond ability	8
Loose rock coming away when climbing	9
Abseiling—i.e., roping down a cliff or rock face	7
Climbing alone or without belays	7
Caught in avalanche	4
Extremely severe weather	3
Fall when aiding in rescue	3
Inadequate equipment	3
Fall due to piton coming out when climbing	2
Crag-fast	1
Cave-diving	1
Sleep-walking	1
Multiple causes, indefinite, unknown, etc.	50

TABLE I.—*Analysis of Mountain Accidents in 1963 and 1964*

Accidents	Wales		Lake District		Pennines		Scotland		Other Areas		Totals	
	1963	1964	1963	1964	1963	1964	1963	1964	1963	1964	1963	1964
Totals	44	36	70	55	16	15	28	50	2	3	160	159
Injured	39	31	65	49	11	11	25	37	1	2	141	130
Fatal	5	5	5	6	5	4	3	13	1	1	19	29
Walking	15 (3)*	11 (2)	47 (4)	34 (1)	3 (1)	9 (3)	6 (1)	21 (4)	1 (1)	1 (1)	72	76
Climbing	29 (2)	23 (3)	23 (1)	21 (5)	7 (3)	2	9 (2)	12 (5)	1	2	68	60
Caving	—	—	—	—	6 (1)	4 (1)	—	—	—	—	7	4
Unknown	—	—	—	—	—	—	13	17 (4)	—	—	13	17

* Figures in parentheses indicate fatal injuries.

184

Besides dealing with these accidents rescue teams have been called out on many occasions to search for missing persons and rescue crag-fast walkers, who have eventually been rescued or found uninjured. These cases are excluded from the accident statistics.

Comments

It will be noted that these mountain accidents are distributed more or less equally between walkers and climbers. Head injuries make up about a quarter of the total. If climbers could be persuaded to wear helmets similar to industrial helmets many of these injuries, which are so often fatal, might be avoided. The British Mountaineering Council and the International Committee for Alpine Rescue (I.K.A.R.) and the Union Internationale des Associations d'Alpinisme (U.I.A.A.) are investigating suitable designs for a climber's helmet.

Fractures usually involve the lower limbs. A double Thomas splint is most often used for immobilizing these fractures. As both legs are secured in this splint it is very useful when the patient has to be lowered down a cliff during the rescue and it is essential for him to be firmly strapped in. Kramer wire splinting is used at some posts as a first-aid splint and inflatable jet splints which fit over the boot and trousers have recently been found effective and comfortable.

Cases of exposure and exhaustion continue to occur in increasing numbers, especially among the young. Recently valuable papers on these problems have appeared in both the medical and mountaineering literature. Pugh (1964), Edholm (1963), and Edholm *et al.* (1964) have given details of the importance of maintaining the body core heat and stressed the need for adequate clothing, insulation, and food to prevent exposure, and how it should be treated by the proper application of adequate heat.

The Mountain Rescue Committee keeps the equipment used under review and considers suggestions and modifications which might prove helpful. Experience has shown that simplicity of design and good wearing and keeping qualities are of great importance in all equipment to be used in mountain-rescue kits.

The administration of morphine by first-aid personnel has been amply justified in practice by the experience of hundreds of persons injured in the hills. As in mine injuries, where morphine may be administered by lay persons, six, 12, or more hours may elapse after injury before the injured person is admitted to hospital. Strong warnings are given to users of official mountain-rescue equipment against the use of morphine in cases of head injury or unconsciousness, and to date no case of overdosage or misuse has been recorded.

Radiotelecommunication, now that transistorized instruments are available, is being used at busy posts by some rescue teams. The R.A.F. have used walkie-talkies in the field for many years. A national scheme is being formed between the G.P.O., the Services, and the Mountain Rescue Committee so that radio communications may be linked on a wide basis rather than confined locally.

A wider review of mountain rescue may be obtained from the R.A.F. handbook *Mountain Rescue,* and from the handbook of the Mountain Rescue Committee (1965).

Much remains to be done to reduce the numbers of accidents on the hills, and many improvements in mountain rescue are required, but a host of willing volunteers in mountain-rescue teams, civilian and R.A.F., British Red Cross and St. John's Ambulance workers, and innumerable climbers, walkers, and police have given and continue to give help to those ill or injured in the mountains.

Summary

Increasing numbers of people are visiting the mountainous areas of Great Britain and about 200 accidents occur there each year. Mountain rescue services are organized by the Mountain Rescue Committee formed from mountaineering clubs in this country and from other outdoor organizations. An analysis of injuries due to mountain accidents in 1963 and 1964 shows that half the persons injured were 21 years old or less ; injuries were equally distributed between walkers and climbers. Exposure and exhaustion occur frequently and could be avoided by climbers having better clothing and food supplies.

The author is grateful to his colleagues on the Mountain Rescue Committee for assistance in the preparation of this paper, to Mr. H. K. Hartley, Secretary and Statistician, for statistical information, to Mr. O. O. Cowpe, Assistant Equipment Officer and Issuing Officer for Morphia, and Mr. A. I. L. Maitland, Equipment Officer for Scotland, for reading the manuscript, and to Mr. A. S. Pigott, O.B.E., Chairman, for much helpful advice.

REFERENCES

Brit. med. J., 1964, 2, 1279.
Edholm, O. G., Duff, D. G., Berkeley, J. S., Murray, W. H., and Blain, R. (1964). *British Mountaineering Council Circular,* November, 1964.
—— (1963). *The Climber,* October, p. 23. Maxwell, Castle Douglas.
Mountain Rescue Committee (1965). *Mountain Rescue and Cave Rescue.* Mountain Rescue Committee, Hill House, Cheadle Hulme, Cheshire.
Pugh, L. G. C. (1964). *Lancet,* 1, 1210.
Royal Air Force (1953). *Mountain Rescue,* May, A.M. 299. Air Ministry, London.

Mechanisms of Death in Shallow-Water Scuba Diving

E. M. COOPERMAN, M.D.,* J. HOGG, M.D., M.Sc. and
W. M. THURLBECK, M.B., M.C.Path.

THE first practical forms of SCUBA (self-contained underwater breathing apparatus) equipment were designed for escape from sunken submarines and were modified during World War II for use in clearing mines from ports and in clandestine military operations, e.g., "frogmen". These Scubas were oxygen re-breather gear with CO_2 absorbent canisters and they have not gone into civilian use. The open-circuit compressed air gear now so widely popular stems from the work of Cousteau and Gagnan in France during and just after the German occupation. Initial interest in the development of Scuba arose then partly because of the military implications. After the Second World War, when efficient compressed-air gear became available, there was a rapidly expanding interest in Scuba diving as a sport, and at present there are an estimated eight million divers in the U.S.A. alone. The sport has serious hazards, but even in the best medical centres there are few physicians who have adequate understanding of the physiological changes

which may be incurred while diving, or knowledge of the wide range of complications that
may result.

CASE REPORT

R.W., a 21-year-old male flying cadet, was
brought to the Emergency Department of the Royal
Victoria Hospital, Montreal, about four hours after
losing consciousness during a Scuba diving exercise
in a standard-sized indoor swimming pool. It was
reported that this young diver had been in excellent
health; his annual chest radiograph and physical
examination were within normal limits.

Observers at the pool-side had noted that the
diver rose to the surface without his equipment,
expired forcibly and then fell back into the water.
He was brought to the pool-side by another diver
approximately one minute later and rushed to the
local infirmary, where he was found to be comatose
and to have pulmonary edema; a blood pressure
of 80/0 was recorded.

On arrival at the Royal Victoria Hospital, the
patient had regained consciousness and had an
accurate memory of events up to the time of entering the pool. He complained of severe retrosternal
chest pain and shortness of breath. On examination
pulmonary edema was noted and was confirmed by
radiography. An electrocardiogram indicated a
massive anteroseptal myocardial infarction. Neurological examination revealed complete right-sided
hemiparesis and absent right abdominal reflexes.
Management was symptomatic, but his condition
deteriorated and terminally the patient was oliguric.
Vigorous resuscitation efforts were undertaken for
some two hours, but although initially successful,
eventually failed. He was pronounced dead approximately 23 hours after the accident had occurred.

The Scuba equipment used by the diver was
found at the bottom of the pool where he had
apparently discarded it. It was fully examined and
found to be fault-free and in perfect working order.
Reportedly the pool was standard in size with a
9-foot maximum depth.

Autopsy Findings

The body was that of a well-developed muscular
man, measuring 70 ins. in height and weighing 172
lbs. There was marked cyanosis of the lips, ear
lobes and nail beds.

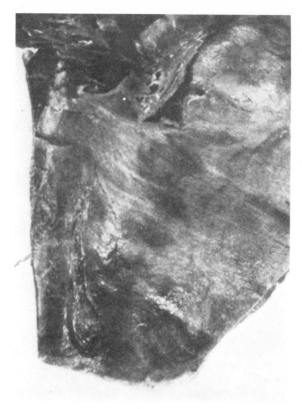

Fig. 1.—The left ventricular muscle is hyperemic with diffuse mottling throughout. (× ¾.)

The heart weighed 450 g. No air could be aspirated from the ventricles. The foramen ovale was closed; the coronary arteries were present in their normal position and distribution. There was no evidence of atherosclerosis in the coronary vessels or aorta. The entire left ventricular wall, including the posterior papillary muscle and the anterior and posterior septum, was mottled (Fig. 1). On microscopic examination the cardiac muscle cells showed fragmentation; the cytoplasm was eosinophilic, with diffuse clumping and granularity. Well-preserved acute inflammatory cells and many erythrocytes lined the interstitial areas of the left ventricular muscle. The lungs were consolidated and firm to palpation. There were no definite signs of pulmonary, interstitial or mediastinal emphysema or pneumothorax. The left lung weighed 1000 g. and the right 1200 g. They were inflated with 20% formalin and cut into sagittal sections after fixation.

189

Microscopic examination of numerous sections showed widespread acute bronchopneumonia, pulmonary edema and hemorrhage (Fig. 2).

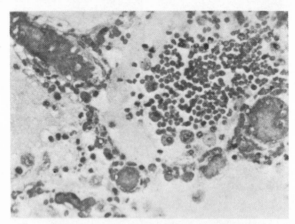

Fig. 2.—Microscopic appearance of the lung: the vessels are markedly congested. Intra-alveolar acute inflammatory cells are prominent. There is some intra-alveolar hemorrhage with diffuse intra-alveolar and interstitial edema. (Hemalum-phloxin-eosin, × 600.)

The left kidney weighed 160 g. and the right 170 g. Marked congestion of the calyces was noted. There was diffuse proximal tubular degeneration and widespread severe acute vascular congestion. The liver weighed 1850 g. and the spleen 360 g.; both were markedly congested. The brain weighed 1500 g. and was diffusely edematous. There was no evidence of cerebral infarction or laminar necrosis.

DISCUSSION

At the time of the accident the patient was engaged in a routine training procedure known as "ditching".[1] In this exercise the diver swims to the pool floor, takes a final breath from his tanks, abandons his equipment and rises to the surface; he then returns and re-dons the equipment. This procedure subjects the unschooled diver to the danger of lung rupture and pneumothorax, or air embolism. It is the diver who takes a full inspiration during the "ditching" procedure that runs the risk of lung rupture because his lungs are already filled to capacity. During training, candidates are advised by their instructors to take a full inspiration at the pool floor, then to rise slowly and exhale

190

throughout the ascent (an action which is contrary to natural inclinations). Lung rupture with its consequences occurs because the regulator valve of Scuba equipment allows air into the lungs at ambient pressure. Thus, pressure in the lungs will exceed atmospheric pressure in proportion to the diver's depth. As he rises towards the surface, ambient pressure decreases and intrapulmonary air expands. This is according to Boyle's law, viz. $P_1 V_1 = P_2 V_2$. Therefore, the pressure volume product at any depth of water will equal the pressure volume product at the water surface. In the case under consideration, the volume at surface,

$$V_2 = \frac{P_1 V_1}{P_2} \text{ or } V_2 = 1.3 \times V \text{ (approx.)}.^*$$

A total lung volume of 5.5 l. (approx.) will expand to a volume of 7 l. (approx.) at the water surface. With the glottis closed, the volume increase in rising from a relatively shallow depth of 9 ft. is thus significant. Moreover, if this increase in volume were prevented by the resistance of the thoracic wall, the pressure in the alveoli would exceed that in the pulmonary vessels by more than 200 mm. Hg.

Apart from ignorance, fear and lack of instruction, the diver may also be subject to the same hazard through focal bronchial obstruction. This may either be congenital or acquired, and although clinically silent and radiologically inapparent, under diving conditions it may produce a ball-valve obstructive lesion. The diver with this deformity will be unable to rid himself of the focal expanding gas volume on rising to the surface and is therefore a candidate for pneumothorax and/or air embolism. There is little doubt that persons who have any special risk of ball-valve obstruction in the form of congenital or acquired lung disease should not engage in Scuba diving.

Presumably, on rising to the surface, increasing volume causes minute alveolar ruptures, and

---

*Using Duffner's chart, the pressure at a depth of 9 ft. is approximately 1.3 x that at the surface.[2]

as the lung volume expands against a closed glottis there is a tendency for air to escape into the left heart circulation. This phenomenon is well illustrated in Duffner's monograph on underwater diving hazards.[2] The target organ, or organs, will depend entirely on the position of the diver at the time the air is released into the left heart circulation. While rather large volumes of air (80 to 100 c.c.) are needed in the right heart circulation to cause serious clinical consequences, small volumes can be fatal in the left heart circulation. As long ago as 1883 it was proved that moderate overinflation of lung parenchyma could result in air embolism without grossly apparent evidence of pneumothorax or severe lung damage.[3, 4] These experiments were carried out on animals and established that as little as 1 c.c. of air in the left heart circulation could result in serious damage to the central nervous system or the myocardium, depending on the position of the animal. Bichat demonstrated that when air is blown into the lung of a living animal, at a pressure no greater than that produced by the maximum expiratory effort of which the animal is capable, air will leave the alveoli and enter the pulmonary capillaries, provided that the pressure is maintained.[3, 6] Neuberger attributed the convulsions of whooping cough to cerebral air embolism from air forced directly into the bloodstream from the alveoli during a paroxysm of coughing.[7, 8]

In the case described in this paper, myocardial circulation was interrupted while the diver was still in the pool. We may assume that the actual occlusion happened as he reached the water surface. It is known from experimental work that coronary occlusion must exist for 15 to 20 minutes before infarction occurs.[5] Air is presumably quickly reabsorbed, and as death took place about one day after the accident occurred one would not expect to be able to aspirate air from the ventricles or to find it in the coronary arteries. No doubt the occlusion must in fact have existed and the air must have remained as an unabsorbed embolic occlusion in the left coronary artery for a length of time sufficient to produce the extensive infarction noted at autopsy. The widespread microscopic hemorrhage seen in most sections of the infarcted heart muscle implies that ultimately the air was completely reabsorbed and total coronary circulation was established. Presumably air emboli caused transient occlusion of the right internal carotid artery which resulted in transient hemiparesis.

THERAPEUTIC IMPLICATIONS

It is a well-known dictum among divers that they are their own best physicians. Medical men, by and large, are ignorant of the physiological hazards of underwater diving and therefore equally ignorant of the rationale of therapy. Besides air embolism, the following major hazards of diving have been described: drowning, usually secondary to physical exhaustion; the bends and asphyxia, suffocation or strangulation.[9] Squeeze or barotrauma is a hazard of the traditional helmet diver. It should not occur in Scuba diving unless the gear misfunctions, except locally as in face-mask squeeze affecting the eyes, and external ear squeeze from a closely fitting hood. Narcosis from CO_2 and oxygen poisoning are only remote possibilities with the modern equipment now used by most amateurs. Carbon monoxide and other toxic gases may get into the tanks, but probably overbreathing is a more frequent cause of clouded consciousness. Examples of the more minor hazards of Scuba diving include otitis (ruptured drum) and sinus barotrauma, disc herniation (from weight of gear in the dry), chilling and abrasions. The mechanisms involved are fully explained in the U.S. Navy Diving Manual.[9] Logical treatment in the case of air embolism is to shrink and dissolve the embolus. Recompression treatment should be put into effect at the very earliest suspicion of air embolism. Prevention of this hazard should be the prime objective of divers, who should be fully familiar with the physiological changes occurring in diving ascent and descent.

Summary A previously healthy young male cadet engaged in shallow water Scuba

193

"ditching" exercises lost consciousness and died approximately 24 hours later. Having taken a full inspiration at the pool floor, the diver neglected to exhale; on rising to the surface, the intrapulmonary air expanded in accordance with Boyle's Law. Under such conditions, often in the absence of visible lung rupture, very small amounts of air may be forced into the left heart circulation and result in air embolism with serious clinical consequences. One of these complications, well illustrated in the case described, is "dysbaric cerebral embolism". In addition, transient occlusion of the coronary circulation in this patient led to extensive myocardial infarction. With the expanding interest in Scuba diving as a sport, it is important that physicians should acquaint themselves with the physiological changes that occur in diving, the potential hazards of this activity and the rationale of therapy.

REFERENCES

1. WAITE, C. L. et al.: Dysbaric cerebral air embolism. In: Underwater physiology: proceedings of the 3rd symposium on underwater physiology, Washington, D.C., March 23-25, 1966, edited by C. J. Lambertsen, The Williams & Wilkins Company, Baltimore, 1967, p. 205.
2. DUFFNER, G. J.: Clin. Sympos., 12: 75, 1960.
3. BEHNKE, A. R.: U.S. Nav. Med. Bull., 30: 177, 1932.
4. EWALD, J. R. AND KOBERT, R.: Pflueger Arch. Ges. Physiol., 31: 360, 1883. Cited by Van Allen, C. M., Hrdina, L. S. and Clark, J.: Arch. Surg. (Chicago), 19: 568, 1929. Cited by Behnke, A. R.: U.S. Nav. Med. Bull., 30: 180, 1932.
5. BLUMGART, H. L., GILLIGAN, D. R. AND SCHLESINGER, M. J.: Amer. Heart J., 22: 374, 1941.
6. BICHAT: Cited by Beneke, R.: Verh. Dtsch. Ges. Path., 16: 263, 1913. Cited by Van Allen, C. M., Hrdina, L. S. and Clark, J.: Arch. Surg. (Chicago), 19: 568, 1929. Cited by Behnke, A. R.: U.S. Nav. Med. Bull., 30: 180, 1932.
7. VAN ALLEN, C. M., HRDINA, L. S. AND CLARK, J.: Arch. Surg. (Chicago), 19: 567, 1929.
8. NEUBURGER, K.: Klin. Wschr., 4: 113, 1925. Cited by Van Allen, C. M., Hrdina, L. S. and Clark, J.: Arch. Surg. (Chicago), 19: 569, 1929.
9. United States Ships Bureau (Navy), Defense Department: U.S. Navy diving manual, pt. 1 (NAVSHIPS 250-538), Superintendent of Documents, U.S. Government Printing Office, Washington, July 1963.

POWER-BOAT INJURIES TO SWIMMERS

DENNIS C. PATERSON, F.R.C.S., F.R.A.C.S., AND JOHN G. SWEENEY, M.Ch.(Orth.), F.R.C.S., F.R.A.C.S.

THE increasing popularity of water-skiing in recent years has resulted in a considerable number of accidents to swimmers and skiers. Many fractures have occurred, including a fracture-dislocation of the cervical spine. There have also been various types of soft-tissue injuries, ranging from severe abdominal injuries to simple strains of joints. The increasing number of motor-boats themselves, however, constitutes a very real hazard to both swimmers and skiers.

In January, 1968, four children suffered severe injuries to their limbs from accidents with power-boats. Two of these children were admitted to the Adelaide Children's Hospital, Inc.

REPORTS OF CASES

CASE 1.—A boy, aged 13 years, was on a surf-board with three other boys when a speed-boat swung round, catching his left leg and throwing him into the water. His left leg was caught in the propeller of the motor-boat. He sustained extensive lacerations to his leg below the knee (Figure 1), and in addition severely comminuted fractures of the tibia, os calcis and metatarsal bones—all as a result of cuts with the propeller blades (Figure 2).

Extensive *débridement* of the wounds was carried out, and, amazingly, at operation all tendons and nerves were found to be intact. The tibial fracture was stabilized with a screw, and the wounds were closed with extensive split skin grafting. Two weeks later the patient required further skin grafting.

195

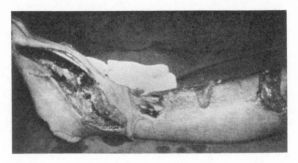

FIGURE 1: Case 1: Showing extensive lacerations to the leg of a boy, aged 13 years.

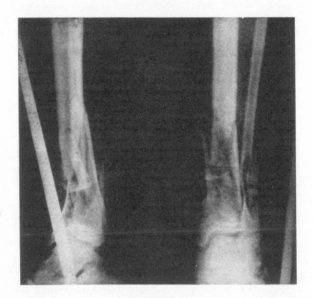

FIGURE 2: Case 1: Showing a severely comminuted fracture of the tibia.

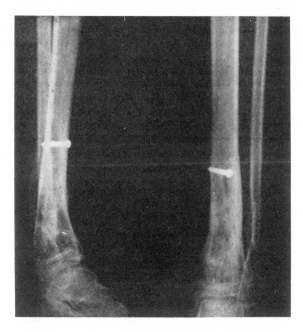

FIGURE 3: Case 1: Showing the fractured tibia to be united, with some backward angulation.

Six months later he was walking with a pronounced limp on the left side, he had regained 20° of plantar flexion of his ankle joint but no dorsiflexion, and his fractured tibia had united with some backward angulation (Figure 3). He is likely to be left with a limp and marked restriction of movement of his ankle joint.

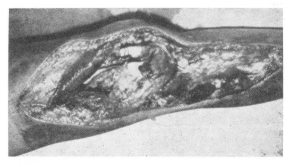

FIGURE 4: Case 2: Showing extensive laceration of the thigh and leg of a girl, aged 11 years; involvement of the knee joint in this laceration is seen.

CASE 2.—This girl, aged 11 years, jumped off a jetty and was run over by a motor-boat which caught her left leg in the propeller, and she suffered severe lacerations to her leg. There was a large, gaping laceration (Figure 4) extending from the mid-thigh to the lower third of the tibia on the

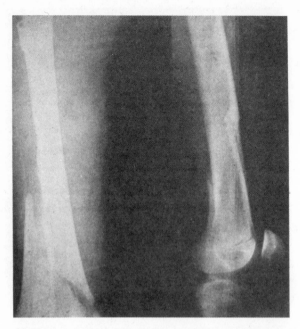

FIGURE 5 : Case 2 : Showing the fracture of the lower end
of the femur extending into the intercondylar region.

anterior surface of the leg. Clinically and radiologically, a
large longitudinal fracture of the lower end of the femur
was present, extending into the intercondylar area (Figure
5). This was stabilized by the insertion of three screws. The
knee joint was extensively involved in the injury and was
reconstituted, and a repair of the patellar tendon and quadriceps muscle was carried out. The leg was splinted in a
Thomas splint. The patient developed some skin necrosis, and
subsequently had extensive skin grafting to try to cover the
defect. However, some of the tibia was left exposed in the
lower end of the wound, and subsequently she had a
sequestrum removed and a further skin graft.

After two months, she was allowed up in a weight-reliev-
ing caliper. One month later, she was allowed to start
bending her knee, but developed a pathological fracture and
required further splintage.

Seven months after the injury, the patient is walking well
out of her caliper, has 10° of flexion of the left knee joint,
and already has about half an inch of shortening of her left
leg because of premature fusion of the lower femoral
epiphysis (Figure 6). It is unlikely that she will regain much
movement in her left knee as a result of this injury. She will
have extensive cosmetic disabilities from the scars, requiring
plastic surgery (Figure 7). She will also require epiphysio-
desis of the lower femoral epiphysis of her good leg, to prevent a discrepancy in her leg lengths.

The other two children injured were reported in *The
Advertiser* (Adelaide) as follows:

A ten year old boy lost his left arm, and his fourteen
year old sister's left leg was severely injured when a

198

power boat, driven by their father, ran over them on a
dam in northern New South Wales. The father stated

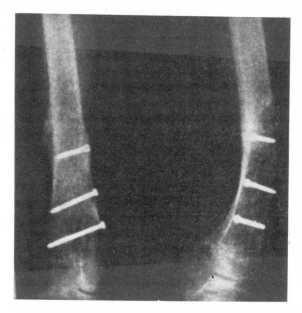

FIGURE 6: Case 2: Showing union of the fracture of the
femur with three transverse screws, and also premature
fusion of the lower femoral epiphysis.

that he was watching another boat which was towing
skiers and was not aware of his own children playing
on rubber floats.

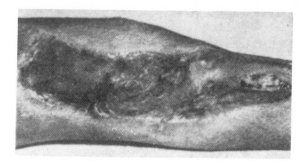

FIGURE 7: Case 2: Showing extensive cosmetic scarring
of the leg from the injury.

HOW CAN THESE ACCIDENTS BE PREVENTED?

In South Australia there are regulations under the

Harbours Act, 1936-1955, for the control of vessels 200 ft. or less in overall length. These regulations are essential for the control of power-boats. This is to ensure the protection of the occupants, and also of skiers and swimmers in the water. A power-boat can be just as difficult to control as a car, and yet no licence is necessary to drive one.

The insistence on the presence of an observer over the age of 16 years in the boat, and a ski rope 70 ft. in length, are good safeguards against accidents; yet these severe accidents have occurred.

Some form of insurance is essential to protect swimmers and skiers in case accidents occur. Water-ski clubs have insurance policies, and it is therefore in the interest of water-skiers to join a club for their own protection.

While it is essential for swimmers to be as careful as possible, and to make certain that they are nowhere near motor-boats, it is suggested that a greater effort should be made to alert the drivers of these motor-boats to the damage they may cause from lack of observance of the regulations under the Act.

REHABILITATION OF THE INJURED ATHLETE

C. ROY RYLANDER, PH.D.

A college trainer or a high school coach who finds it necessary to handle his own training problems in addition to his coaching or a local physician who helps out with a high school program will find that his duties in the training area are divided into three fields: the prevention of injuries, the treatment of injuries, and the rehabilitation of the injured athlete. In a successful athletic program, the essential ingredient is complete mutual confidence and cooperation of coach, trainer and physician, with the physician being the final authority regarding the first aid, treatment and rehabilitation of the injured athlete.[1]

Prevention, treatment, and rehabilitation are each important parts of the overall injury care program. Great strides have been made in the area of prevention regarding equipment, conditioning and the discouragement of tactics endangering the players. Similarly, sports medicine has made great advances in treatment including prompt, accurate and complete examination and diagnosis of the degree of the injury, and the development and use of physical therapy modalities sometimes in

201

conjunction with the use of drugs such as muscle relaxants, anti-inflammatory cortico-steroids, and oral enzymes.[2]

An integral part of the treatment of any injury is rehabilitation, but it is in this area where coaches, trainers and physicians have most neglected the athletes. In too many instances, an injured athlete is pronounced recovered and free of symptoms and immediately returned to full duty, with or without supportive wrappings, only to become re-injured very shortly thereafter. It is in the area of rehabilitation where the greatest contribution toward our injury care program can still be made. Of all the modalities available for the treatment of athletic injuries, probably the most effective is active exercise.[3,4] This includes isometric and isotonic exercise programs.

O'Donoghue[1] lists five concepts of treatment to govern the rehabilitation program.

They are:
1. Treatment must be prompt to minimize severity and disability.
2. The best treatment possible must be used.
3. Expediency is to be avoided.
4. Competitive ability should be restored.
5. The goal must be complete recovery.

Rehabilitation

The passage of time is not a measure of rehabilitation.[5] Rehabilitation is a fundamental part of the treatment of any injury and deals primarily with the restoration of muscle function. Treatment should therefore be based not only upon the evaluation of the bones and the joints concerned, but equally upon consideration of the status of the muscle.[6] Athletic injuries are in large part peculiar to the performance requirements for each particular sport. The injuries are characterized by recurrent exposure to injury-producing circumstances, making re-injury a strong possibility. In addition, the athlete is subject to the strains of all-out performance and therefore requires repair and rebuilding of injured parts beyond that ordinarily required for normal or sedentary activity.[1]

Restoration of muscle function is accomplished by an exercise program which is based on an evaluation of muscle strength, muscle flexibility or elasticity, and the ability of the muscle to relax.

Muscle function and strength will be increased if the exercises are repeated often enough and with sufficient intensity to exceed easy performance in each exercise period; if the exercise sessions are on a regular basis and for a long total period of time; and if the exercises performed are identical.

Ideally, muscle strength of the injured side should be graded[7] and compared with the uninjured side before strengthening exercises are prescribed. This is of value in demonstrating dramatically to the coach and player concerned just how much strength has been lost, in measuring progress, and in setting up a progressive exercise program of sufficient intensity.

Athletes today spend a great deal of time and effort readying themselves for a sport season by developing strength, endurance, flexibility and agility. The same principles apply to the redevelopment of these qualities in muscles weakened through injury. Repeated usage of a small or low weight develops endurance; few repetitions with high resistance develops strength. It should be pointed out that it is possible to cause pain and a decrease in strength with an overly-ambitious program.

Karpovich[8] and Hooks,[9] in their texts on weight training in athletics, present general rules for determining how much weight to use. For exercises involving the upper extremities and the chest, Karpovich and Murray advocate starting out with a weight which can be handled for a maximum of eight repetitions. One repetition is then added for each training period until twelve repetitions are reached. At this point five to ten pounds are added with the number of repetitions starting again at eight with the same upward progression. For exercising the legs and lower back a weight is chosen which can be handled a maximum of ten repetitions. One repetition is added each training period until the number of repetitions reaches 15 to 18, at which time ten or twenty pounds are added and the cycle restarted. Klein[10] has developed a progressive resistive program for strengthening the quadriceps and hamstrings of which some exercises have a maximum of one to four repetitions.

Often because of pain and weakness following injury, active and passive assistive exercises[11] without weights, with gravity eliminated, or simply against gravity are required initially. Active resistive exercises have several advantages. Strength of a muscle or group of muscles varies at the various positions in the joint range. Therefore, in order to complete a range of movement the use of weights must necessarily be limited to the maximum weight that can be lifted through the full range. This is generally much less than the weight which can be handled in the sector of maximum capacity. In addition, manual resistance and assistance enable strengthening as well as stretching of tight muscles in one exercise period. This is not possible with weights[6]. At no time in the rehabilitation of muscle or joint injuries should forcible manipulations be used; this only causes additional tissue damage and delay in recovery.

Both isotonic and isometric exercises may be used. Isotonic exercise becomes isometric exercise when the last possible repetition is reached, and has the additional advantage of developing the cardio-vascular-respiratory system. Isometrics, when done properly, have the advantage of being able to develop specifically the particularly weak sectors in the range of motion of a joint. Bender[12] uses this exercise technique in his multiple-angle testing method for evaluation and development of muscle strength, but this requires rather expensive equipment.

I personally favor isotonic exercise. The trainer and the player then know the status of strength on any given day and do not need expensive equipment to determine this. In addition, the player seems to develop more confidence through participation in the isotonic program, and this is important.

The use of electrical muscle stimulation, ultrasound, the application of ice or ethyl chloride, and the use of muscle relaxant and anti-inflammatory drugs, when and where applicable as determined by a physician, may be helpful in the early stages of restoration of function.

Return to Unlimited Activity

The question arises, "When is an injured player to be allowed to return to his sport without restriction?" In general the answers to this are when the range of motion of the affected part is normal, when the injured side is at least approximately as strong as the uninjured side, and when, with special strapping or protection, the athlete is symptom free.[5] Equally important is that when this point is reached, the athete's confidence has been fully restored. Re-injury is then largely a matter of coincidence.

At the University of Delaware,[13] for example, a boy with a sprained knee is deemed sufficiently recovered when he can fully extend the knee, with a 60-pound load, ten times in forty seconds and run a tight figure "8" at full speed (while taped) without pain or feeling of weakness.

Fortunately, with injured athletes we are

dealing with young people who are in otherwise good health, have good conditioning, are highly motivated, and possess a natural disposition for maximum restoration, all of which enables them to return to their sport in the shortest possible time.

Summary

Great strides have been made in the areas of prevention of athletic injuries and in the care and treatment of those injuries which inevitably occur. It is in the area of rehabilitation of the injured athlete where there is much room for improvement in our injury care program. Exercise is probably the most effective treatment modality, and exercise prescribed should use the techniques of De Lorme's progressive resistance exercise. Minimum levels of muscle strength for each particular muscle group, especially for knee, shoulder and low back injuries, should be obtained before an athlete is allowed to return to play without restriction. The passage of time is not a measure of rehabilitation.

REFERENCES

1. O'Donoghue, D. H.: A doctor talks about injuries to athletes. Journal of Health, Phys. Ed. and Rec. 31:8, p. 22, 1960.
2. Donoho, C. R., and Rylander, C. R.: Proteolytic enzymes in athletic injuries. Del. Med.Jour. 34:168, 1962.
3. Novich, M. M.: Physical therapy in treatment of athletic injuries. Tex. St. Jour. Med. 61:672, 1965.
4. Jokl, E.: The Scope of Exercisein Rehabilitation. p. 128, 1964.
5. Kraus, H.: Physical conditioning and the prevention of athletic injury. Proc. First Nat. Conf. on the Med. Aspects of Sports. AMA. p. 98, Nov. 30, 1959.
6. Kraus, H.: Evaluation and treatment of muscle function in athletic injury. Amer. Jour. Surg. 98:353, 1959.
7. Rusk, H. A.: Rehabilitation Medicine. Chapter 1, 2, 3, 1965.
8. Karpovich, P. V., and Murray, J.: Weight training in athletics. p. 214, 1956.
9. Hooks, G.: Application of Weight Training to Athletics. pp. xiii, 254.
10. Klein, K. K.: Progressive resistive exercise and its utilization in the recovery period following knee injury. The Jour. of Assoc. for Phys. and Ment. Rehab. 10:3, p. 94, 1956.
11. Krusen, F H.: Physical Medicine and Rehabilitation for the clinician. Chap. 5, 38, 1951.
12. Bender, J. A., Kobes, F. J., Kaplan, H. M., and Pierson, J. K.: Strengthening muscles and preventing injury with a controlled program of isometric exercises. Jour. Health, Phys. Ed. and Rec., 35:57, 1964.
13. Donoho, C. R., and Rylander, C. R.: The football knee—a general plan for rehabilitation of a sprained knee. Del. Med. Jour. 38:20, 1966.

A Clinic for Athletic Injuries

Mr P H Newman, Mr J P S Thomson,
Dr J M Barnes and Dr T M C Moore

A clinic for athletic injuries was started at the Middlesex Hospital twenty-one years ago. Dr Ben Woodard was the first post-war accident officer and, having a special connexion with the AAA, became involved in the treatment of athletic injuries at the time of training for the Olympic Games held in London in 1948. He quickly built up a personal reputation by his dedication to the welfare of athletes and his understanding of their temperament and requirements.

When he left it was difficult to foresee how such an arrangement could continue, but the new accident officer was asked to make himself available three mornings a week to see athletes. That the clinic has continued demonstrates its potential value in this special sphere of accident work.

A general hospital is not an ideal place for seeing athletic and other sporting injuries, in fact it is a most inappropriate place if the athlete is to maintain the tempo and the competitive motivation of peak achievement. An accident

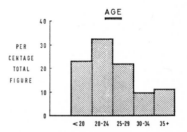

Fig 1 *Age distribution of the series*

or casualty department cannot afford to give priority or special understanding to the athlete, and in the orthopædic departments the waiting time for consultation often runs into several weeks. Proper treatment of an athlete among the acutely ill, the chronically sick, and the geriatric is not practical.

Since Dr Woodard left the Middlesex Hospital, there has been no attempt to attract, in any way, the acute injury. The hospital is neither geographically nor temperamentally disposed to

207

work as a field unit. But there is a permanent arrangement whereby an athlete can have comparatively prompt advice and attention by a medical officer of registrar status who understands what is required. If special advice or in-patient treatment is necessary, the patient can be referred to the next clinic conducted by one of the supervising consultant orthopædic surgeons.

Some recent figures of patients who have attended the clinic may be of interest. It was decided to carry out a retrospective survey of the notes of all new patients attending the clinic during the years 1958, 1959, 1967 and 1968 (until September 30). The yearly figures were 397, 610, 410 and 430 respectively, and these made a series total of 1,847 new patients. From this total figure we derived the following information:

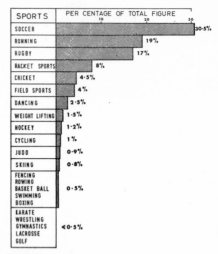

Fig 3 *Sports*

DELAY IN ATTENDING CLINIC

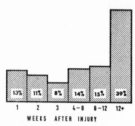

Fig 2 *Delay in attending the clinic after injury or onset of symptoms*

Sports (Fig 3): Patients injured while involved in soccer, running, Rugby, and racket sports account for almost 75% of the total series.

Injuries: Table 1 shows the anatomical distribution of the injuries. Corrigan (1968) classified

Table 1
Injuries in 1,847 new patients:
Middlesex Hospital Clinic for athletic injuries

	%
Knee	31
Ankle	14
Muscle	14
Back and neck	9
Shoulder	5
Foot	5
Tendocalcaneus	3
Elbow	3
Stress fractures	2
Hand	2
Others	12

Age (Fig 1): The majority of the patients were, as expected, under 30 years of age, but it is interesting to note that the youngest patient in the series was a boy swimmer of 9 who had a rotator cuff lesion, and the oldest patient was a runner of 75 who had pulled his left hamstring muscles.

Delay in attendance (Fig 2): 68% of the patients attended the clinic three or more weeks after their injury or the onset of their symptoms. That only 13% of the patients came to the clinic within seven days of injury clearly demonstrates its function as a clinic for persistent and difficult problems, and not for the routine first-aid treatment of injury.

athletic injuries into three groups: direct injuries, where the part is injured by a direct knock or blow; indirect injuries, where the cause is other than direct external violence; over-use syndromes, where the only predisposing cause is the patient's athletic activity. This series has been classified into these three groups: 15% had direct injuries, 57% indirect injuries, and 28% had over-use syndromes. As would be expected, the proportions of these three groups varied with different

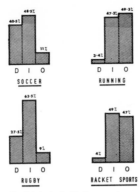

Fig 4 *Injuries in the four most common sports classified.*
D=direct injury. I=indirect injury. O=over-use syn-
dromes

Table 2
Treatments for athletic injuries (Middlesex Hospital)

	%
Physiotherapy (heat, ice, exercises, frictions, balance boards)	67
Injection (with hydrocortisone and 1 % lignocaine hydrochloride)	18
Immobilization (crepe bandage, elastoplast strapping, pressure bandage, plastic splints, plaster of paris, &c.)	15
Reassurance and advice	10
Operative	2
Others (including rest and manipulative treatment)	5

The total exceeds 100%, as some patients received more than one
form of treatment

sports. Fig 4 illustrates the findings in the four
most common sports of the series.

Treatment: Table 2 shows the treatment given.
In studying the different ways of treating patients
in this clinic, it must be remembered that they are
late cases which have frequently not responded to
the usual first-line methods. The majority of the
patients had physiotherapy in some form. The
Department of Physiotherapy is a training school,
and this has the advantage of providing sufficient
senior students to take special small classes at
certain times exclusively for rehabilitation of
athletes.

REFERENCE
Corrigan A B (1968) *Hosp. Med.* **2**, 1328

AUTHOR INDEX

KEY-WORD TITLE INDEX